PEDIATRICS, CHILD AND ADOLESCENT HEALTH

PEDIATRICS AND ADOLESCENT HEALTH

RECENT INTERNATIONAL RESEARCH

PEDIATRICS, CHILD AND ADOLESCENT HEALTH

JOAV MERRICK - SERIES EDITOR

NATIONAL INSTITUTE OF CHILD HEALTH AND HUMAN DEVELOPMENT, MINISTRY OF SOCIAL AFFAIRS, JERUSALEM

Pediatrics and Adolescent Health: Recent International Research
Joav Merrick and Mohammed Morad (Editors)
2022. ISBN: 978-1-68507-490-6 (Hardcover)

Why Do Children Die? Selective Perspectives on Thanatology in Pediatrics
Donald E Greydanus, Dustin C Rowland and Joav Merrick (Editors)
2022. ISBN: 978-1-68507-461-6 (Hardcover)

Caring for the Newborn: A Comprehensive Guide for the Clinician. Second Edition
Donald E Greydanus, Shibani Kanungo, Cheryl Dickson and Joav Merrick (Editors)
2021. ISBN: 978-1-53619-462-3 (Hardcover)
2021. ISBN: 978-1-53619-801-0 (e-book)

Adolescence: International Aspects of Psychological Stress
Supa Pengpid, Karl Peltzer and Joav Merrick (Editors)
2021. ISBN: 978-1-53618-341-1 (Hardcover)
2021. ISBN: 978-1-53619-696-2 (e-book)

Pediatric and Adolescent Sexuality and Gynecology: Principles for the Primary Care Clinician, Second Edition
Hatim A Omar, Donald E Greydanus, Dilip R Patel and Joav Merrick (Editors)
2021. ISBN: 978-1-53619-340-4 (Hardcover)
2021. ISBN: 978-1-53619-607-8 (e-book)

Building Children and Youth for the Future: Some International Aspects
Joav Merrick, Ariel Tenenbaum and Hatim A Omar (Editors)
2021. ISBN: 978-1-53618-806-6 (Hardcover)
2021. ISBN: 978-1-53619-017-5 (e-book)

Building Children and Youth for the Future: Some International Aspects
Joav Merrick, Ariel Tenenbaum Hatim A Omar (Editors)
2021. ISBN: 978-1-53618-806-6 (Hardcover)
2021. ISBN: 978-1-53619-017-5 (e-book)

Tropical Pediatrics: a Public Health Concern of International Proportions, 3rd Edition
Richard R Roach, Donald E Greydanus, Dilip R Patel, and Joav Merrick (Editors)
2021. ISBN: 978-1-53618-604-8 (Hardcover)
2021. ISBN: 978-1-53618-928-5 (e-book)

Childhood and Adolescence: Perspectives of Pain
Donald E Greydanus and Joav Merrick (Editors)
2020: ISBN 978-1-53618-416-7 (Hardcover)
2020: ISBN 978-1-53618-633-8 (e-book)

Adolescence: International Aspects of Interpersonal and Self-Directed Violence
Supa Pengpid, Karl Peltzer and Joav Merrick (Editors)
2020. ISBN: 978-1-53618-066-4 (Softcover)
2020. ISBN: 978-1-53618-067-1 (e-book)

School Health in Asia and Africa
Supa Pengpid, Karl Peltzer and Joav Merrick (Editors)
2020. ISBN: 978-1-53617-868-5 (Hardcover)
2020. ISBN: 978-1-53617-869-2 (e-book)

Chronic Disease and Disability: The Pediatric Liver
Donald E Greydanus, Ransome Eke, Orhan Atay and Joav Merrick (Editors)
2020. ISBN: 978-1-53617-750-3 (Hardcover)
2020. ISBN: 978-1-53617-751-0 (e-book)

Chronic Disease and Disability: The Pediatric Heart, Second Edition
Donald E Greydanus, Premchand Anne, John D. Rowlett and Joav Merrick (Editors)
2020. ISBN: 978-1-53617-656-8 (Hardcover)
2020. ISBN: 978-1-53617-657-5 (e-book)

Adolescence: Behavioural Risk Factors of Non-Communicable Diseases
Supa Pengpid, Karl Peltzer and Joav Merrick (Editors)
2020. ISBN: 978-1-53617-704-6 (Hardcover)
2020. ISBN: 978-1-53617-705-3 (e-book)

Adolescence in Curaçao
Soraya Verstraeten, Supa Pengpid, Karl Peltzer and Joav Merrick (Editors)
2020. ISBN: 978-1-53617-522-6 (Softcover)
2020. ISBN: 978-1-53617-523-3 (e-book)

Building Youth for the Future: Suicide Prevention Aspects
Hatim A. Omar and Joav Merrick (Editors)
2019. ISBN: 978-1-53615-799-4 (Hardcover)
2019. ISBN: 978-1-53616-565-4 (e-book)

Vaccine: Measles and Rubella Vaccination Experience in Zambia
Mazyanga L. Mazaba-Liwewe, Seter Siziya and Joav Merrick (Editors)
2019. ISBN: 978-1-53615-799-4 (Hardcover)
2019. ISBN: 978-1-53615-800-7 (e-book)

The Boko Haram Terror: Adversary to the Wellbeing of Nigerian Kids
Miracle A. Adesina, Kehinde K. Kanmodi and Joav Merrick (Editors)
2019. ISBN: 978-1-53615-443-6 (Softcover)
2019. ISBN: 978-1-53615-444-3 (e-book)

Chronic Disease and Disability: Pediatric Obesity Perspectives
Marisha Agana, Donald E. Greydanus, Manmohan K. Kamboj and Joav Merrick (Editors)
2019. ISBN: 978-1-53615-240-1 (Hardcover)
2019. ISBN: 978-1-53615-241-8 (e-book)

Substance Use Disorders in Adolescents and Young Adults: A Manual for Pediatric and Primary Care Clinicians. Second Edition
Donald E. Greydanus, Gabriel Kaplan, Dilip R. Patel and Joav Merrick (Editors)
2019. ISBN: 978-1-53615-359-0 (Hardcover)
2019. ISBN: 978-1-53615-360-6 (e-book)

Building Youth for the Future: A Path towards Suicide Prevention
Hatim A. Omar and Joav Merrick (Editors)
2018. ISBN: 978-1-53613-768-2 (Hardcover)
2018. ISBN: 978-1-53613-769-9 (e-book)

Soft Skills and Aspirations in Chinese Children and Youth
Daniel T.L. Shek, Janet TY Leung and Joav Merrick (Editors)
2018. ISBN: 978-1-53614-092-7 (Hardcover)
2018. ISBN: 978-1-53614-093-4 (e-book)

Childhood and Adolescence: Tribute to Emanuel Chigier, 1928-2017
Joav Merrick (Editor)
2018. ISBN: 978-1-53613-574-9 (Hardcover)
2018. ISBN: 978-1-53613-574-9 (e-book)

Child Health and Human Development Yearbook 2017
Joav Merrick (Editor)
2018. ISBN: 978-1-53613-628-9 (Hardcover)
2018. ISBN: 978-1-53613-629-6 (e-book)

Child and Adolescent Health Yearbook 2017
Joav Merrick (Editor)
2018. ISBN: 978-1-53613-594-7 (Hardcover)
2018. ISBN: 978-1-53613-595-4 (e-book)

Chronic Disease and Disability: The Pediatric Gastrointestinal Tract
Donald E Greydanus, Orhan Atay and Joav Merrick (Editors)
2018. ISBN: 978-1-53612-948-9 (Hardcover)
2018. ISBN: 978-1-53612-949-6 (e-book)

Multiple Sclerosis in Children and Adolescents
Hatim Omar and Joshua Chalkley (Editors)
2018. ISBN: 978-1-53612-979-3 (Hardcover)
2018. ISBN: 978-1-53612-980-9 (e-book)

Childhood and Adolescence: Tribute to Emanuel Chigier, 1928-2017
Joav Merrick (Editor)
2018. ISBN: 978-1-53613-574-9 (Softcover)
2018. ISBN: 978-1-53613-575-6 (e-book)

Chronic Disease and Disability: The Pediatric Lung
Donald E Greydanus, Myrtha M Gregoire-Bottex, Kevin W Cates and Joav Merrick (Editors)
2018. ISBN: 978-1-53613-577-0 (Hardcover)
2018. ISBN: 978-1-53613-578-7 (e-book)

Bicycles: Helmet Use of Adolescents at Independent Schools
Ronald Chow, Michael Borean, Drew Hollenberg, Jaclyn Viehweger, Tharani Anpalagan and Anna Rzepka (Editors)
2017. ISBN: 978-1-53612-458-3 (Hardcover)
2017. ISBN: 978-1-53612-459-0 (e-book)

Positive Youth Development: Long Term Effects in a Chinese Program
Daniel TL Shek, Cecilia MS Ma, Janet TY Leung and Joav Merrick (Editors)
2017. ISBN: 978-1-53612-539-9 (Hardcover)
2017. ISBN: 978-1-53612-540-5 (e-book)

Adolescence: Bicycle and Helmet Use of Adolescents and Young Adults
Ronald Chow and Joav Merrick (Editors)
2017. ISBN: 978-1-53612-039-4 (Hardcover)
2017. ISBN: 978-1-53612-060-8 (e-book)

Suicide: A Global View on Suicidal Ideation among Adolescents
Mazyanga L. Mazaba, Seter Siziya and Joav Merrick (Editors)
2017. ISBN: 978-1-53611-788-2 (Hardcover)
2017. ISBN: 978-1-53611-799-8 (e-book)

Children and Youth: Post-Traumatic Stress Disorder and Motor Vehicle Crashes
Donald E. Greydanus, Roger W. Apple, Kathryn White, and Joav Merrick (Editors)
2017. ISBN: 978-1-53611-102-6 (Hardcover)
2017. ISBN: 978-1-53611-255-9 (e-book)

Child and Adolescent Health Yearbook 2016
Joav Merrick (Editor)
2017. ISBN: 978-1-53610-948-1 (Hardcover)
2017. ISBN: 978-1-53610-957-3 (e-book)

Child Health and Human Development Yearbook 2016
Joav Merrick (Editor)
2017. ISBN: 978-1-53610-946-7 (Hardcover)
2017. ISBN: 978-1-53610-958-0 (e-book)

Chronic Disease and Disability: The Pediatric Kidney
Donald E Greydanus, Vimal Master Sankar Raj, and Joav Merrick (Editors)
2016. ISBN: 978-1-63483-793-4 (Hardcover)
2015. ISBN: 978-1-63483-809-2 (e-book)

Child and Adolescent Health Yearbook 2015
Joav Merrick (Editor)
2016. ISBN: 978-1-63484-512-0 (Hardcover)
2016. ISBN: 978-1-63484-543-4 (e-book)

Child Health and Human Development Yearbook 2015
Joav Merrick (Editor)
2016. ISBN: 978-1-63484-513-7 (Hardcover)
2016. ISBN: 978-1-63484-544-1 (e-book)

Pain Management Yearbook 2015
Joav Merrick (Editor)
2016. ISBN: 978-1-63484-515-1 (Hardcover)
2016. ISBN: 978-1-63484-545-8 (e-book)

Children and Childhood: Some International Aspects
Joav Merrick (Editor)
2016. ISBN: 978-1-63484-587-8 (Hardcover)
2016. ISBN: 978-1-63484-594-6 (e-book)

Children and Adolescents: Future Challenges
Daniel TL Shek, Tak Yan Lee, and Joav Merrick (Editors)
2016. ISBN: 978-1-63484-616-5 (Hardcover)
2016. ISBN: 978-1-63484-627-1 (e-book)

Adolescence: Positive Youth Development Programs in Chinese Communities
Daniel TL Shek, Florence KY Wu, Janet TY Leung, and Joav Merrick (Editors)
2016. ISBN: 978-1-63484-044-6 (Hardcover)
2016. ISBN: 978-1-63484-677-6 (e-book)

Growing Up in the Middle East: The Daily Lives and Well-Being of Israeli and Palestinian Youth
Yossi Harel-Fisch, Ziad Abdeen and Miriam Navot
2016. ISBN: 978-1-63484-746-9 (Hardcover)
2016. ISBN: 978-1-63484-765-0 (e-book)

Sexuality: Some International Aspects
Joav Merrick and Donald E Greydanus (Editors)
2016. ISBN: 978-1-63484-707-0 (Hardcover)
2016. ISBN: 978-1-63484-719-3 (e-book)

Chronic Disease and Disability: The Pediatric Heart
Donald E Greydanus, Devika Malhotra and Joav Merrick (Editors)
2016. ISBN: 978-1-63484-828-2 (Hardcover)
2016. ISBN: 978-1-63484-842-8 (e-book)

Diabetes Mellitus: Childhood and Adolescence
Manmohan K Kamboj, Donald E Greydanus and Joav Merrick (Editors)
2016. ISBN: 978-1-53610-095-2 (Hardcover)
2016. ISBN: 978-1-53610-104-1 (e-book)

Chronic Disease and Disability: Abuse and Neglect in Childhood and Adolescence
Donald E Greydanus, Vincent J Palusci and Joav Merrick (Editors)
2016. ISBN: 978-1-53610-129-4 (Hardcover)
2016. ISBN: 978-1-53610-142-3 (e-book)

Clinical Aspects of Psychopharmacology in Childhood and Adolescence, Second Edition
Donald E Greydanus, Joseph L Calles, Jr, Dilip R Patel, Ahsan Nazeer and Joav Merrick (Editors)
2016. ISBN: 978-1-53610-241-3 (Hardcover)
2016. ISBN: 978-1-53610-253-6 (e-book)

Chronic Disease and Disability: The Pediatric Pancreas
Donald E Greydanus, Manmohan K Kamboj and Joav Merrick (Editors)
2016. ISBN: 978-1-53610-055-6 (Hardcover)
2016. ISBN: 978-1-53610-065-5 (e-book)

A Pediatric Resident Pocket Guide: Making the Most of Morning Reports
Arthur N Feinberg
2015. ISBN: 978-1-63482-141-4 (Softcover)
2015. ISBN: 978-1-63482-186-5 (e-book)

Child and Adolescent Health Yearbook 2014
Joav Merrick (Editor)
2015. ISBN: 978-1-63482-162-9 (Hardcover)
2015. ISBN: 978-1-63482-206-0 (e-book)

Tropical Pediatrics: A Public Health Concern of International Proportions Second Edition
Richard R Roach, Donald E Greydanus, Dilip R Patel and Joav Merrick (Editors)
2015. ISBN: 978-1-63463-381-9 (Hardcover)
2015. ISBN: 978-1-63463-404-5 (e-book)

Child and Adolescent Health Issues (A Tribute to the Pediatrician Donald E Greydanus)
Joav Merrick (Editor)
2015. ISBN: 978-1-63463-574-5 (Hardcover)
2015. ISBN: 978-1-63463-576-9 (e-book)

Child Health and Human Development Yearbook 2014
Joav Merrick (Editor)
2015. ISBN: 978-1-63482-163-6 (Hardcover)
2015. ISBN: 978-1-63482-207-7 (e-book)

Behavioral Pediatrics, 4th Edition
Donald E Greydanus, Dilip R Patel, Helen D Pratt, Joseph L Calles Jr, Ahsan Nazeer and Joav Merrick (Editors)
2015. ISBN: 978-1-63483-027-0 (Hardcover)
2015. ISBN: 978-1-63483-052-2 (e-book)

Disability, Chronic Disease and Human Development
Joav Merrick
2015. ISBN: 978-1-63483-029-4 (Hardcover)
2015. ISBN: 978-1-63483-057-7 (e-book)

Caribbean Adolescents: Some Public Health Concerns
Cecilia Hegamin-Younge and Joav Merrick (Editors)
2015. ISBN: 978-1-63483-341-7 (Hardcover)
2015. ISBN: 978-1-63483-343-1 (e-book)

Adolescence and Health: Some International Perspectives
Joav Merrick (Editor)
2015. ISBN: 978-1-63483-791-0 (Hardcover)
2015. ISBN: 978-1-63483-808-5 (e-book)

Youth Suicide Prevention: Everybody's Business
Hatim A Omar (Editor)
2015. ISBN: 978-1-63483-786-6 (Softcover)
2015. ISBN: 978-1-63483-820-7 (e-book)

Human Developmental Research: Experience from Research in Hong Kong
Daniel TL Shek, Cecilia Ma, Yu Lu and Joav Merrick (Editors)
2014. ISBN: 978-1-62808-166-4 (Hardcover)
2013. ISBN: 978-1-62808-167-1 (e-book)

School, Adolescence and Health Issues
Joav Merrick, Ariel Tenenbaum and Hatim A Omar (Editors)
2014. ISBN: 978-1-62948-702-1 (Hardcover)
2014. ISBN: 978-1-62948-707-6 (e-book)

Adolescence and Sexuality: International Perspectives
Joav Merrick, Ariel Tenenbaum and Hatim A Omar (Editors)
2014. ISBN: 978-1-62948-711-3 (Hardcover)
2014. ISBN: 978-1-62948-724-3 (e-book)

Child and Adolescent Health Yearbook 2013
Joav Merrick (Editor)
2014. ISBN: 978-1-63117-658-6 (Hardcover)
2014. ISBN: 978-1-63117-668-5 (e-book)

Adoption: The Search for a New Parenthood
Gary Diamond and Eva Arbel
2014. ISBN: 978-1-63117-710-1 (Hardcover)
2014. ISBN: 978-1-63117-713-2 (e-book)

Adolescence: Places and Spaces
Myra F Taylor, Julie Ann Pooley and Joav Merrick (Editors)
2014. ISBN: 978-1-63117-847-4 (Hardcover)
2014. ISBN: 978-1-63117-850-4 (e-book)

Child Health and Human Development Yearbook 2013
Joav Merrick (Editor)
2014. ISBN: 978-1-63117-939-6 (Hardcover)
2013. ISBN: 978-1-63117-958-7 (e-book)

Born into this World: Health Issues
Donald E Greydanus, Arthur N Feinberg, and Joav Merrick (Editors)
2014. ISBN: 978-1-63321-667-9 (Hardcover)
2014. ISBN: 978-1-63321-669-3 (e-book)

Caring for the Newborn: A Comprehensive Guide for the Clinician
Donald E Greydanus, Arthur N Feinberg and Joav Merrick (Editors)
2014. ISBN: 978-1-63321-760-7 (Hardcover)
2014. ISBN: 978-1-63321-781-2 (e-book)

Environment and Hope: Impoving Health, Reducing AIDS and Promoting Food Security in the World
Leslie Rubin and Joav Merrick (Editors)
2014. ISBN: 978-1-63321-772-0 (Hardcover)
2014. ISBN: 978-1-63321-782-9 (e-book)

Pain Management Yearbook 2013
Joav Merrick (Editor)
2014. ISBN: 978-1-63117-944-0 (Hardcover)
2014. ISBN: 978-1-63117-959-4 (e-book)

Pediatric and Adolescent Dermatology: Some Current Issues
Donald E Greydanus, Arthur N Feinberg and Joav Merrick (Editors)
2014. ISBN: 978-1-63321-853-6 (Hardcover)
2014. ISBN: 978-1-63321-863-5 (e-book)

Adolescence and Behavior Issues in a Chinese Context
Daniel TL Shek, Rachel CF Sun, and Joav Merrick (Editors)
2013. ISBN: 978-1-62618-614-9 (Hardcover)
2013. ISBN: 978-1-62618-692-7 (e-book)

Advances in Preterm Infant Research
Jing Sun, Nicholas Buys and Joav Merrick
2013. ISBN: 978-1-62618-696-5 (Hardcover)
2013. ISBN: 978-1-62618-775-7 (e-book)

Child Health and Human Development: Social, Economic and Environmental Factors
Leslie Rubin and Joav Merrick (Editors)
2013. ISBN: 978-1-62948-166-1 (Hardcover)
2013. ISBN: 978-1-62948-169-2 (e-book)

Children, Violence and Bullying: International Perspectives
Joav Merrick, Isack Kandel and Hatim A Omar (Editors)
2013. ISBN: 978-1-62948-342-9 (Hardcover)
2013. ISBN: 978-1-62948-345-0 (e-book)

Chinese Adolescent Development: Economic Disadvantages, Parents and Intrapersonal Development
Daniel TL Shek, Rachel CF Sun and Joav Merrick (Editors)
2013. ISBN: 978-1-62618-622-4 (Hardcover)
2013. ISBN: 978-1-62618-694-1 (e-book)

Chronic Disease and Disability in Childhood
Joav Merrick
2013. ISBN: 978-1-62808-865-6 (Hardcover)
2013. ISBN: 978-1-62808-868-7 (e-book)

Environmental Health Disparities in Children: Asthma, Obesity and Food
Leslie Rubin and Joav Merrick (Editors)
2013. ISBN: 978-1-62948-122-7 (Hardcover)
2013. ISBN: 978-1-62948-135-7 (e-book)

Environmental Health: Home, School and Community
Leslie Rubin and Joav Merrick (Editors)
2013. ISBN: 978-1-62948-155-5 (Hardcover)
2013. ISBN: 978-1-62948-158-6 (e-book)

Guidelines for the Healthy Integration of the Ill Child in the Educational System: Experience from Israel
Yosefa Isenberg
2013. ISBN: 978-1-62808-350-7 (Hardcover)
2013. ISBN: 978-1-62808-353-8 (e-book)

Internet Addiction: A Public Health Concern in Adolescence
Artemis Tsitsika, Mari Janikian, Donald E Greydanus, Hatim A Omar and Joav Merrick (Editors)
2013. ISBN: 978-1-62618-925-6 (Hardcover)
2013. ISBN: 978-1-62618-959-1 (e-book)

Playing with Fire: Children, Adolescents and Firesetting
Hatim A Omar, Carrie Howell Bowling and Joav Merrick (Editors)
2013. ISBN: 978-1-62948-471-6 (Softcover)
2013. ISBN: 978-1-62948-474-7 (e-book)

Promotion of Holistic Development of Young People in Hong Kong
Daniel TL Shek, Tak Yan Lee and Joav Merrick (Editors)
2013. ISBN: 978-1-62808-019-3 (Hardcover)
2013. ISBN: 978-1-62808-040-7 (e-book)

University and College Students: Health and Development Issues for the Leaders of Tomorrow
Daniel TL Shek, Rachel CF Sun and Joav Merrick (Editors)
2013. ISBN: 978-1-62618-586-9 (Hardcover)
2013. ISBN: 978-1-62618-612-5 (e-book)

Break the Cycle of Environmental Health Disparities: Maternal and Child Health Aspects
Leslie Rubin and Joav Merrick (Editors)
2013. ISBN: 978-1-62948-107-4 (Hardcover)
2013. ISBN: 978-1-62948-133-3 (e-book)

Child and Adolescent Health Yearbook 2012
Joav Merrick (Editor)
2012. ISBN: 978-1-61942-788-4 (Hardcover)
2012. ISBN: 978-1-61942-789-1 (e-book)

Child Health and Human Development Yearbook 2011
Joav Merrick (Editor)
2012. ISBN: 978-1-61942-969-7 (Hardcover)
2012. ISBN: 978-1-61942-970-3 (e-book)

Child and Adolescent Health Yearbook 2011
Joav Merrick (Editor)
2012. ISBN: 978-1-61942-782-2 (Hardcover)
2012. ISBN: 978-1-61942-783-9 (e-book)

Tropical Pediatrics: A Public Health Concern of International Proportions
Richard R Roach, Donald E Greydanus, Dilip R Patel, Douglas N Homnick and Joav Merrick (Editors)
2012. ISBN: 978-1-61942-831-7 (Hardcover)
2012. ISBN: 978-1-61942-840-9 (e-book)

Child Health and Human Development Yearbook 2012
Joav Merrick (Editor)
2012. ISBN: 978-1-61942-978-9 (Hardcover)
2012. ISBN: 978-1-61942-979-6 (e-book)

Developmental Issues in Chinese Adolescents
Daniel TL Shek, Rachel CF Sun and Joav Merrick (Editors)
2012. ISBN: 978-1-62081-262-4 (Hardcover)
2012. ISBN: 978-1-62081-270-9 (e-book)

Positive Youth Development: Theory, Research and Application
Daniel TL Shek, Rachel CF Sun and Joav Merrick (Editors)
2012. ISBN: 978-1-62081-305-8 (Hardcover)
2012. ISBN: 978-1-62081-347-8 (e-book)

Understanding Autism Spectrum Disorder: Current Research Aspects
Ditza A Zachor and Joav Merrick (Editors)
2012. ISBN: 978-1-62081-353-9 (Hardcover)
2012. ISBN: 978-1-62081-390-4 (e-book)

Positive Youth Development: A New School Curriculum to Tackle Adolescent Developmental Issues
Hing Keung Ma, Daniel TL Shek and Joav Merrick (Editors)
2012. ISBN: 978-1-62081-384-3 (Hardcover)
2012. ISBN: 978-1-62081-385-0 (e-book)

Transition from Pediatric to Adult Medical Care
David Wood, John G Reiss, Maria E Ferris, Linda R Edwards and Joav Merrick (Editors)
2012. ISBN: 978-1-62081-409-3 (Hardcover)
2012. ISBN: 978-1-62081-412-3 (e-book)

PEDIATRICS, CHILD AND ADOLESCENT HEALTH

PEDIATRICS AND ADOLESCENT HEALTH

RECENT INTERNATIONAL RESEARCH

JOAV MERRICK
AND
MOHAMMED MORAD
EDITORS

nova
Medicine & Health
New York

CONTENTS

INTRODUCTION

In: Pediatrics and Adolescent Health ISBN: 978-1-68507-490-6
Editors: J. Merrick and M. Morad

Chapter 1

SMOKING AND OTHER ISSUES IN CHILDHOOD AND ADOLESCENCE

Joav Merrick[1-4,*], MD, MMedSci, DMSc and Mohammed Morad[2,5,6], MD, FRCP

[1]Department of Pediatrics, Mt Scopus Campus, Hadassah Hebrew University Medical Center, Jerusalem, Israel
[2]National Institute of Child Health and Human Development, Jerusalem, Israel
[3]Kentucky Children's Hospital, University of Kentucky, Lexington, Kentucky, USA
[4]Center for Healthy Development, School of Public Health, Georgia State University, Atlanta, USA
[5]Clalit Health Services
[6]Department of Family Medicine, Division of Community Health, Faculty of Health Sciences, Ben Gurion University of the Negev, Beer Sheva, Israel

[*] Corresponding Author's E-mail: jmerrick@zahav.net.il.

Abstract

About one in four youths used a tobacco product during the past 30 days. By school level this is approximately three in ten high school students and one in eight middle school students. Since 2014, e-cigarettes have been the most commonly used tobacco product among youths. It is reasonable to assume that many of the young smokers are practicing this habit while with friends or at parties, exposing their friends and peers to hazardous passive smoking, which is also the case for smaller children exposed to their parental smoking. Smoking is just one important public health issue in childhood and adolescence, but there are many other issues in this period of our development. In this book we have gathered some recent research on children and youth from various places around the world on many other topics than smoking which we hope will be of interest to the reader.

Introduction

Tobacco was first consumed by pre-Columbian American natives. These American Indians grew tobacco and developed ceremonial as well as medical uses for smoking this Trojan horse product. It was introduced to Europe in the 16th century and was popularized by such figures as the French diplomat, Jean Nicot (1530-1600), for whom nicotine was named. Use of tobacco was increased after the United States Civil War (1861-1865) by the overwhelming acceptance of tobacco grown in North Carolina and Virginia. Cyclopean and predatory promotion by the tobacco corporations and the movie industry increased the use of tobacco in the 20th century until the historic release of the first report of the Surgeon General's Advisory Committee on Smoking and Health on January 11, 1964. This report by Luther L Terry, MD identified the severe adverse effects of tobacco as a tenebrous product that first addicts the victim and later kills him or her with cancer or heart disease. The United States government has launched a major, on-going campaign since then to educate the unwary public to the major dangers of tobacco resulting in far fewer Americans addicted to tobacco in the 21st century in contrast to the previous centenary (1).

Despite current knowledge of the adverse nature of tobacco, the premature deaths of over 400,000 Americans each year from tobacco (5 million worldwide premature deaths), this product continues to be grown and promoted with the aid of governments, societies, and the tobacco enterprise. In its 31st publication on tobacco by the US Surgeon General's office, the government concluded that the threat on the health of youth and young adults remains real and unremitting (1). Indeed this plant turns our children, youth and young adults into helpless victims who blindly smoke this chemical until they prematurely die years later from its relentless and well-known complications.

THE NATIONAL YOUTH TOBACCO SURVEY IN 2019

The United States National Youth Tobacco Survey (NYTS) has been conducted periodically during 1999–2009, but annually since 2011 providing data on estimates of tobacco product use among the youth of America. It is the only nationally representative survey of US middle school (grades 6–8) and high school (grades 9–12) students focused on tobacco product use and associated factors. From 1999 to 2018 the surveys had been conducted via paper and pencil questionnaires, but in 2019 it was administered for the first time in schools using electronic data collection methods (2).

The Center for Disease Control and Prevention (CDC) and the US Food and Drug Administration (FDA) analyzed data from the 2019 NYTS. Overall, 19,018 questionnaires were completed and weighted to represent approximately 27.0 million students. On the basis of self-reported grade level, this included 8,837 middle school questionnaires (11.9 million students) and 10,097 high school questionnaires (15.0 million students); 84 questionnaires with missing information on grade level were excluded from school-level analyses (2).

TOBACCO USE IN 2019

About one in four youths (23.0%) had used a tobacco product during the past 30 days. By school level, this represented approximately three in ten high school students (31.2%) and approximately one in eight middle school students (12.5%). Since 2014, e-cigarettes have been the most commonly used tobacco product among youths. Importantly, more than half of current youth tobacco product users reported seriously thinking about quitting all tobacco products in 2019.

It is reasonable to assume that many of the young smokers are practicing this habit while with friends or at parties, exposing their friends and peers to hazardous passive smoking.

CONCLUSION

In 2019, the prevalence of cigarette smoking among youths was the lowest ever found by these surveys since 1999. An estimated 5.8% of high school students and 2.3% of middle school students reported current cigarette smoking in 2019, compared with 28.5% of high school students and 9.2% of middle school students in 1999. However, youths are using various other tobacco products, most notably e-cigarettes (2), which turned out to have possible devastating consequences as recently reported (3). The surveys are important public health tools to understand trends over time and target and guide prevention efforts to reduce harmful health impact on our youth.

In this book we have gathered some recent research on children and youth from various places around the world on many other topics that we hope will be of interest to the reader.

REFERENCES

[1] Donald E. Greydanus, Gabriel Kaplan, Dilip Patel and Joav Merrick, eds. Substance use disorders in adolescents and young adults: A manual for pediatric and primary care clinicians, Second edition. New York: Nova Science, 2019:XIX-XXIX.

[2] Wang TW, Gentzke AS, Creamer MR, Cullen KA, Holder-Hayes E, Sawdey MD, et al. Tobacco product use and associated factors among middle and high school students: United States, 2019. MMWR 2019; 68(12):1–22.

[3] King JL, Reboussin BA, Merten JW, Wiseman KD, Wagoner KG, Sutfin EL. Negative health symptoms reported by youth e-cigarette users: Results from a national survey of US youth. Addict Behav 2020;104:106315. doi: 10.1016/j.addbeh.2020.106315.

SECTION ONE: CHILD HEALTH ISSUES

In: Pediatrics and Adolescent Health ISBN: 978-1-68507-490-6
Editors: J. Merrick and M. Morad

Chapter 2

ADVERSE CHILDHOOD EXPERIENCES AND CHILD HEALTH INSURANCE COVERAGE

Kandice Lacci**, *Katelin Beals*, *Melissa Knutsen*, *Ryan Scales* and *Larissa R Brunner Huber*, *PhD

University of North Carolina at Charlotte,
College of Health and Human Services,
Department of Public Health Sciences, Charlotte,
North Carolina, USA

ABSTRACT

Previous research indicates that adverse childhood experiences (ACEs) are associated with worse health outcomes for both children and adults, compared to children who are not exposed to ACEs. ACEs are identified as: sexual, physical, and emotional abuse; parent/guardian divorce; and living in a household with a parent/guardian who has a mental illness, abuses alcohol or drugs, was incarcerated, or was/is involved in intimate partner violence. Objective: The present chapter

---

* Corresponding Author's E-mail: Klacci@uncc.edu.

aims to explore the relationship between exposure to ACEs and child health insurance coverage and sufficiency of insurance coverage to meet the child's needs. Study group: The study used data from the 2011-2012 United States National Survey of Children's Health (N = 95,677). Methods: ACEs, insurance coverage, and sufficiency of coverage were self-reported by the guardian of the child. Multivariate logistic regression was conducted to determine the association between ACEs and the two outcomes, child health insurance coverage and sufficiency of insurance coverage to meet the needs of the child. Results: After adjustment, children with ACEs had increased odds of being uninsured as compared to children without ACEs (1 ACE: OR = 1.48; 95% CI = 1.19-1.85 & = 2 ACEs: OR = 1.56; 95% CI = 1.25-1.96). There was no statistically significant association between ACEs and sufficiency of coverage (1 ACE: OR = 1.30; 95% CI=0.81, 2.11 & = 2 ACEs: OR = 0.80; 95% CI = 0.50, 1.27). Conclusions: This study reveals a potential disparity in child health insurance coverage associated with ACEs. These findings provide support for improving health insurance coverage among children with ACEs.

INTRODUCTION

In 2017, an estimated 34 million children in the United States encountered at least one adverse childhood experience (ACE) (1). ACEs are defined as traumatic events that can occur throughout a child's development, often resulting in high amounts of prolonged stress and deleteriously impact well-being (2). Events classified as ACEs include: sexual, physical, and emotional abuse; parent/guardian divorce; and living in a household with a parent/guardian who has a mental illness, abuses alcohol or drugs, was incarcerated, or was/is involved in intimate partner violence (3). Children who have experienced ACEs are subject to high amounts of prolonged stress, or toxic stress, which can increase the risk for health problems during childhood and adulthood compared to individuals who have not faced ACEs (4). The 1998 CDC-Kaiser ACE study found that childhood exposure to adverse events significantly increased the odds for seven of the leading causes of death in the United States. Specifically, individuals in the study who had four or more ACEs had increased odds of ischemic heart disease (AOR = 2.2; 95% CI = 1.3,

3.7), cancer (AOR = 1.9; 95% CI = 1.3, 2.7), and stroke (AOR = 2.4; 95% CI = 1.3, 4.3) as adults (5). In addition, a 2017 meta-analysis reported an increased risk for depression (OR = 4.40; 95% CI = 3.54, 5.46), problematic drug use (OR = 10.22; 95% CI = 7.62, 13.71), heavy alcohol use (OR = 2.20; 95% CI = 1.74, 2.78) and interpersonal or self-directed violence (OR = 8.10; 95% CI = 5.87, 11.18) in individuals who had experienced four or more ACEs as compared to individuals who experienced fewer than four ACEs (6).

Recent studies have also examined the effects of childhood trauma on the child's current health status. A 2017 cross-sectional study assessed whether combinations of ACEs have different effects on child health outcomes (7). After controlling for covariates, including race, age, gender, family income, number of children in the home, family structure, and the mother's education and health status, children with multiple ACEs had a statistically significant increased risk of parent-reported poor child health (OR = 2.39; 95% CI: 1.36, 4.20). Children with both parental mental illness and poverty also had an increased risk of parent-reported poor child health (OR = 2.95; 95% CI: 2.21, 3.93). These findings were consistent with past studies that suggested that cumulative ACE scores are highly associated with numerous child health outcomes (7).

The increased risk of adverse health outcomes in adulthood, including alcohol and drug dependence, tobacco use, and mental illnesses, among those who have experienced ACEs as children, indicates an increased need for health care utilization. However, in 2016, 5.1% of children in the United States were uninsured (8, 9). A 2017 study that assessed the relationship between ACEs and health care utilization among adults in the United States revealed that individuals who had experienced ACEs had decreased odds of being insured in adulthood (OR = 0.56-0.79) (10). Furthermore, all ACEs, except for sexual abuse, were associated with reduced odds of having received a routine check-up in the last year (10). Without health insurance, a primary care doctor visit costs on average $160 (11). Children who have experienced ACEs and do not have health insurance are not likely to obtain the health care services they need because of the high prices. This can lead to more child deaths, low quality of life, and reduced life expectancy (6).

There has been an increased focus over the last twenty years on the impact of ACEs on adult and child health outcomes. While a previous study evaluated the association between ACEs and adult health insurance coverage, little is known about the relationship between exposure to ACEs and child health insurance coverage (10). The purpose of this study was to explore the ACEs- child health insurance coverage association as well as the potential association between ACEs and whether the parents felt the insurance coverage was adequate for their child's health needs.

OUR STUDY

This study utilized data from the 2011-2012 National Survey of Children's Health (NSCH), which is an annual cross-sectional telephone survey (9). Data collection with the NSCH is reviewed by the US Census Bureau and does not undergo an external review by an Institutional Review Board (8); however the data is protected and treated with sensitivity and was used ethically within this study. The survey was administered in the United States to households that had at least one child, under the age of 18 years, residing in the home between February 2011 and June 2012. Study participants were selected using stratification by state and phone type (cell phone or landline), in addition to clustering for families with more than one child living in a household. In each state, random digit dialing of cell phone and landlines was based off wire-center location and area codes, respectively. The survey collected complete data on 95,677 children (landline response rate: 38.2% and cell phone response rate: 15.5%) (12).

During the survey, trained interviewers administered a 33-minute questionnaire in English, Mandarin, Cantonese, Vietnamese, or Spanish with the guidance of a computer-assisted telephone interviewing system. (12). The survey was administered to the parent or guardian with the most knowledge about the child's health. The questionnaire inquired about demographics, family characteristics, physical and mental health of the child, and environmental and community factors that impact health. Individuals who lacked data on ACE exposure (n = 15,722), child health insurance coverage (n = 166), or sufficiency of coverage (n = 4,879) were excluded from this study. Thus, 95,677 individuals remained for analysis.

During the telephone survey, parents or guardians were asked nine questions regarding ACE exposure, including whether the child was exposed to: (i) financial hardship, (ii) parent/guardian divorce, (iii) death of a parent/guardian, (iv) incarceration of a parent/guardian, (v) domestic violence, (vi) neighborhood violence, (vii) living in a household with an individual who suffers from a mental disorder, (viii) substance abuse, and (ix) racism. If a parent or guardian answered "yes" to any of these nine questions, the child was considered to have that ACE. The number of ACEs that each child experienced was then added to obtain an overall ACE score. These scores were categorized as follows: 0 (referent), 1, and = 2.

There were two main outcomes of interest: child health insurance coverage and sufficiency of coverage. Data on child health insurance coverage were self-reported by the parent/guardian during the phone interview. If parents/guardians reported "yes" the child was considered to have insurance coverage. When parents/guardians indicated "no" the child was considered to be uninsured. Parents/guardians also self-reported if they felt the insurance plan met the needs of the child. This outcome had five responses: never, sometimes, usually, always, or do not know. Individuals who indicated that they did not know were removed from analysis. Individuals who answered sometimes, usually, or always were classified as "yes" and individuals who answered never were classified as "no." Based on existing literature, several factors were considered as potential confounders, including race/ethnicity of the child (white, black, other), parent/guardian education level, family structure (two parents, single parent, other) parent/guardian employment status, annual household income (<100% FPL, 100-199% FPL, 200-399% FPL, =400% FPL), and the number of children in the household (1, 2, 3, =4) (10). All of these variables were self-reported by the participants and recognized by other studies as related to ACEs and health insurance coverage.

Table 1. Sample characteristics, NCHS 2011-2012 (n = 95,677)

Variable	Frequency *(n)*	Weighted Percent *(%)*
ACEs		
0 ACEs	33,843	39.00
1 ACE	30,998	35.79
≥2 ACEs	21,775	25.14
Insurance status		
Insured	91,471	95.77
Uninsured	4,040	4.23
Sufficient coverage		
Yes	85,932	99.20
No	684	0.79
Age *(years)*		
0-5	27,687	31.97
6-10	23,226	26.81
11-17	35,703	41.22
Sex		
Male	44,533	51.41
Female	42,083	48.59
Race		
White	63,989	74.84
Black	8,461	9.09
Other	13,052	15.27
Family structure		
Two-parent	66,518	78.13
Single-parent	13,368	15.70
Other	5,254	6.17
Total number of children		
1	39,550	41.34
2	35,864	37.48
3	13,870	14.50
≥4	6,393	6.68

Variable	Frequency (n)	Weighted Percent (%)
Parent educational attainment		
<HS degree	10,801	13.15
HS degree	28,026	34.12
>HS degree	43,311	52.73
Parent employment status		
No	8,182	10.68
Yes	68,448	89.32
Poverty level		
<100% FPL	10,079	13.15
100-199% FPL	12,707	16.58
200-399% FPL	24,062	31.4
≥400% FPL	29,782	38.86

Summary statistics were obtained to describe the characteristics of the sample. Logistic regression was used to determine the association between ACE scores and the two outcomes (i.e., insurance coverage and the sufficiency of the coverage) as well as to determine other factors associated with the two outcomes. Multivariate logistic regression was used to calculate adjusted ORs and 95% CIs. If a potential confounder changed the magnitude of the odds ratio by 10% or greater, then the variable was determined to be a confounder of the association between ACE score and the outcome (13). SAS-callable SUDAAN was utilized in all analyses in order to account for the complex sampling design used by NCHS.

OUR FINDINGS

The majority of respondents were white (74.84%), and about half of the study population was female (48.59%; see Table 1). Approximately 70% of the study participants had an annual household income that was above 200% FPL, and 89.3% of parents were employed. Approximately 87% of the sample participants reported parental educational attainment of at least a high school degree or higher.

Among the study participants, 35.8% reported that their child had experienced one ACE, and 25.1% indicated that their child had experienced two or more ACEs. In addition, 95.8% of children in the sample were insured, and 99.2% of survey respondents reported that their child's insurance coverage was sufficient to meet his/her needs.

Table 2. Unadjusted associations between selected characteristics and insurance status and sufficiency of coverage, NCHS 2011-2012 (n = 95,677)

	Insurance status			Sufficient coverage	
	OR	95% CI		OR	95% CI
ACEs					
0 ACEs	1.00	Referent		1.00	Referent
1 ACE	2.33	(1.88, 2.87)		1.85	(1.18, 2.89)
≥ 2 ACEs	2.63	(2.13, 3.25)		1.29	(0.86, 1.92)
Age (years)					
0-5	0.73	(0.60, 0.90)		0.79	(0.50, 1.25)
6-10	0.86	(0.71, 1.04)		0.84	(0.52, 1.37)
11-17	1.00	Referent		1.00	Referent
Sex					
Male	1.00	Referent		1.00	Referent
Female	0.81	(0.69, 0.96)		0.71	(0.48, 1.04)
Race					
White	1.00	Referent		1.00	Referent
Black	0.95	(0.74, 1.23)		1.03	(0.63, 1.66)
Other	1.71	(1.39, 2.11)		2.20	(1.37, 3.52)
Family structure					
Two-parent	1.00	Referent		1.00	Referent
Single-parent	1.09	(0.89, 1.35)		1.17	(0.74, 1.86)
Other	1.18	(0.85, 1.62)		1.60	(0.60, 4.26)
Total number of children					
1	1.00	Referent		1.00	Referent
2	0.72	(0.60, 0.87)		1.05	(0.65, 1.69)
3	0.80	(0.64, 1.02)		1.06	(0.63, 1.79)
≥ 4	1.05	(0.78, 1.41)		1.18	(0.70, 1.98)

	Insurance status			Sufficient coverage	
	OR	95% CI		OR	95% CI
Parental educational attainment					
< HS degree	2.82	(2.29, 3.46)		3.04	(1.86, 4.97)
HS degree	1.34	(1.10, 1.63)		1.53	(1.01, 2.32)
> HS degree	1.00	Referent		1.00	Referent
Parent employment status					
No	1.67	(1.35, 2.07)		2.81	(1.83, 4.29)
Yes	1.00	Referent		1.00	Referent
Poverty level					
< 100% FPL	6.75	(5.01, 9.09)		4.88	(2.91, 8.18)
100-199% FPL	8.46	(6.34, 11.27)		2.70	(1.46, 5.01)
200-399% FPL	3.59	(2.69, 4.80)		2.53	(1.44, 4.45)
≥ 400% FPL	1.00	Referent		1.00	Referent

Table 3. Adjusted odds ratios and 95% CIs of ACEs and insurance status and sufficiency of coverage, NCHS 2011-2012 (n = 95,677)

	Insurance status[1]			Sufficient coverage[2]	
	AOR	95% CI		AOR	95% CI
ACEs (independent variable)					
0 ACEs	1.00	Referent		1.00	Referent
1 ACE	1.48	(1.19, 1.85)		1.30	(0.81, 2.11)
≥ 2 ACEs	1.56	(1.25, 1.96)		0.80	(0.50, 1.27)

[1] adjusted for parent educational attainment and poverty level.

[2] adjusted for parent employment status, parent educational attainment and poverty level.

Before accounting for potential confounders, children who were classified as having one ACE had 2.33 (95% CI= 1.88, 2.87; see Table 2) times the odds of being uninsured as compared to children whose parents reported no ACEs. Children who were classified as having two or more ACEs had 2.63 (95% CI = 2.13, 3.25) increased odds of being uninsured as compared to children whose parents reported no ACEs.

Children whose parents reported one ACE had nearly twice (OR = 1.85; 95% CI = 1.18, 2.89) the odds of having health care coverage that did not meet the child's needs as compared to children whose parents had reported no ACEs, prior to controlling for confounders. In comparison, children whose parents reported at least two ACEs had nearly 30% increased odds (OR = 1.29; 95% CI = 0.89, 1.92) of having health care coverage that does not meet the needs of the child as compared to children whose parents reported no ACEs; however, this finding was not statistically significant. Race, parent educational attainment, parent employment, and poverty level all displayed a statistically significant relationship to both insurance status and adequacy of coverage.

After controlling for the parent educational attainment and poverty level, children who had one ACE had 1.48 (95% CI = 1.19, 1.85) times the odds of being uninsured, and children who had two or more ACEs had 1.56 (95% CI = 1.25, 1.96) times the odds of being uninsured as compared to children who had no ACEs. After adjustment for parent educational attainment, parent employment status and poverty level, there were no statistically significant results for the ACE- insufficient coverage association (1 ACE: OR = 1.30; 95% CI: 0.81, 2.11; >2 ACEs: OR = 0.80; 95% CI: 0.50, 1.27).

CONCLUSION AND DISCUSSION

Although several studies have examined the association between ACEs and health care coverage in adult populations, no studies to our knowledge have explored this association with respect to child health insurance coverage (10). The results of this population-based study indicate that ACEs are associated with child health insurance coverage. After adjusting for confounders, exposure to at least one ACE was associated with increased odds of being uninsured. This is consistent with extant research that examined this relationship among adults (10). In addition, the findings in this study are similar to a prior study that explored the relationship between adult health care coverage and specific ACEs (14). Although ACE exposure was initially associated with increased odds of insufficient insurance coverage, the results failed to remain statistically significant after controlling for confounders. Since no other studies have examined this relationship, these findings cannot be compared to extant data.

This study has several limitations. Since NSCH is a cross-sectional study, causality cannot be determined. Non-differential misclassification of the exposure (ACEs) may have occurred because this information was assessed by parents' self-report. The sensitive nature of ACEs and fear of stigma may have impacted parents' answers to the survey questions. Non-differential misclassification of the outcomes may have also occurred since the sufficiency of coverage and type of health insurance coverage were self-reported by the parents. However, it is unlikely that people reported their insurance status inaccurately. Nonresponse bias was also possible, as the combined landline and cell phone response rate for the survey was 23%; however, sampling weights were adjusted for nonresponse (12).

Despite the limitations of the study, the study had several strengths. The population-based survey that was utilized in this study (NSCH) had a large sample size (n = 95,677 after exclusions). In addition, the sampling design used by NSCH makes the data representative of the United States population, thus enhancing the generalizability of findings. Lastly, interviewer bias is unlikely to have occurred because the interviewers were all trained and followed a detailed survey manual.

This study reveals a potential association between ACEs and health care accessibility. The only other previous study to analyze this association was conducted with an adult population (10). While the majority of parents in this study reported that their child had health insurance coverage, a small percentage of the sample was uninsured (4.23%). This small group of respondents is an important population to target. Increased health care coverage among children with ACEs could allow for more preventative care and decreased risk of chronic disease in adulthood. Increased insurance coverage could also reduce associated medical costs, as many uninsured children with ACEs seek medical care from hospitals. Since ACEs are associated with deleterious health outcomes, increased health insurance coverage could improve health in children who have ACEs. Future research may explore the association between ACEs and specific types of health insurance coverage among children, such as private and government insurance. In addition, future research may examine the association between specific ACEs and child insurance coverage.

ACKNOWLEDGMENTS

The authors declare that they have no conflict of interest. Information used in the study was obtained ethically from the National Survey of Children's Health. This study was conducted in accordance with the 1964 Declaration of Helsinki and its subsequent amendments.

REFERENCES

[1] Robert Wood Johnson Foundation. Traumatic experiences widespread among US youth [Internet]. Princeton, NJ: RWJF, 2017. URL: https://www.rwjf.org/en/library/articles-and-news/2017/10/traumatic-experiences-widespread-among-u-s--youth--new-data-show.html.

[2] Sacks V, Murphey D, Moore K. Adverse childhood experiences: national and state level prevalence. Bethesda, MD: Childtrends.org, 2014. URL: https://www.childtrends.org/wp-content/uploads/2014/07/Brief-adverse-childhood-experiences_FINAL.pdf.

[3] Gilbert LK, Breiding MJ, Merrick MT, Thompson WW, Ford DC, Dhingra SS, et al. Childhood adversity and adult chronic disease. Am J Prev Med 2010;48(3): 345-9.

[4] Center on the Developing Child. Toxic stress. Boston, MA: Harvard University, 2017. URL: https://developingchild.harvard.edu/science/key-concepts/toxic-stress/.

[5] Felitti VJ, Anda RF, Nordenberg D, Williamson DF, Spitz AM, Edwards V, Koss MP, et al. Relationship of childhood abuse and household dysfunction to many of the leading causes of death in adults. Am J Prev Med 1998;14(4):245-58.

[6] Hughes K, Bellis MA, Hardcastle KA, Sethi D, Butchart A, Mikton C, et al. The effect of multiple adverse childhood experiences on health: a systematic review and meta-analysis. Lancet Public Health 2017;2(8):356-66.

[7] Lanier P, Maguire-Jack K, Lombardi B, Frey J, Rose RA. Adverse childhood experiences and child health outcomes: Comparing cumulative risk and latent class approaches. Matern Child Health J 2018;22(3):288-97.

[8] HRSA Center for Integrated Health Solutions. Adverse childhood experiences (ACEs), trauma, and post traumatic stress disorder (PTSD). URL: https://www.integration.samhsa.gov/clinical-practice/trauma

[9] National Center for Health Statistics. Health insurance coverage. Centers for Disease Control and Prevention, 2017. URL: https://www.cdc.gov/nchs/fastats/health-insurance.htm.

[10] Alcalá HE, Valdez-Dadia A, von Ehrenstein OS. Adverse childhood experiences and access and utilization of health care. J Public Health (Oxf) 2018;40(4):684-92.

[11] Johns Hopkins Bloomberg School of Public Health. Primary care visits available to most uninsured but at a high price. Baltimore, MD: Johns Hopkins University, 2015. URL: https://www.jhsph.edu/news/news-releases/2015/primary-care-visits-available-to-most-uninsured-but-at-a-high-price.html.

[12] National Center for Health Statistics. 2011-2012 National Survey of Children's Health. Centers for Disease Control and Prevention, 2013. URL: from http://www.cdc.gov/nchs/slaits/nsch.htm.

[13] Maldonado G, Greenland S. Simulation study of confounder-selection strategies. Am J Epidemiol 1993;138(11):923-36.

[14] Chartier MJ, Walker JR, Naimark B. Separate and cumulative effects of adverse childhood experiences in predicting adult health and health case utilization. Child Abuse Negl 2010;34(6):454-64.

In: Pediatrics and Adolescent Health ISBN: 978-1-68507-490-6
Editors: J. Merrick and M. Morad

Chapter 3

FIFA, BODY COMPOSITION AND PHYSICAL FITNESS AMONG OBESE CHILDREN

***Nur Azis Rohmansyah and Ashira Hiruntrakul**, PhD**
Department of Exercise and Sport Sciences, Faculty of Graduate School, Khon Kaen University, Thailand, Department of Branch of Sport Science, Faculty of Applied Science and Engineer, Khon Kaen University, Nong Khai Campus, Thailand, Department of Physical Education, Universitas PGRI Semarang, Indonesia

ABSTRACT

FIFA 11+ training program has been recognized as an effective means of prevention and treatment for obesity. The FIFA 11+ is a low-to-moderate exercise intensity and with a higher fat oxidation rate than other aerobic exercise intensities. This study aimed to investigate the effect of 12 weeks of the FIFA 11+ training program on body mass index (BMI) and physical fitness among obese adolescents. The study included 20 obese adolescents showed that physical fitness improved (p

* Corresponding Author's E-mail: hashir@kku.ac.th.

= 0.004) and BMI decreased (p = 0.02) significantly before and after intervention. Food intake as a confounding factor was found as a predictor which decreased the BMI (0.74 kcal/day; p = 0.00) better than exercise (0.38 kcal/week; p = 0.176). Obese adolescents and the whole family need to be given an understanding that diet and exercise are not completed when weight loss can be achieved, but calorie restriction must be carried out and become a daily habit.

INTRODUCTION

Worldwide prevalence of obesity has been epidemic (1). Obesity prevalence has increased in all age groups, in particular, in 2018, 21.83% of the Indonesia population was considered obese. Moreover, obesity rates are increasing, with the incidence of obesity in Indonesia increasing from approximately 14.8% in 2013 to 21.8% in 2018 (2). Obesity amongst adolescent may cause low levels of cardiorespiratory fitness (VO2max) and a high percentage of body fat (%BF) are risk factors for many chronic diseases such as diabetes, hypertension, dyslipidemia, and cardiovascular disease (3). Among the different interventions, exercise training has been recognized as an effective means of prevention and treatment for obesity (4). Despite the well-documented benefits of exercise training, many obese individuals do not participate in physical activity citing lack of time as the largest barrier (5). In fact, only 1.5-3.0% of obese adolescents meet the current recommendations of 150 min/week of moderate-intensity continuous training (6), so research is needed to identify practical and effective exercise modalities in this population. Previous exercise training studies in adolescents with obesity have typically designed the exercise intensity at 50% to 85% of the heart rate reserve (7, 8) or at 40% to 80% of maximal oxygen uptake (VO2max) (9).

The FIFA-Medical and Assessment Research Centre (F-MARC) created an advanced version of this training program, the FIFA 11+ program (10). The FIFA 11+ is a low-to-moderate exercise intensity and with a higher fat oxidation rate than other aerobic exercise intensities.

Our team has reported that obese adolescent reached their exercise at 52% VO2max (11). Some researchers have applied the low-to-moderate exercise intensity training to an adolescent with metabolic diseases (12). The main outcomes have included decreased body fat or improved ability to oxidise lipids during exercise in obese adolescent (11). However, to date, there have been no studies that have applied FIFA 11+ exercise training in the obese adolescent. Hence, it is logical to expect FIFA 11+ would be a suitable exercise intensity for obese adolescent people who want to decrease their body fat, as well as improve functional capacity. Therefore, the purpose of the present study was to investigate the effects of FIFA 11+ on body composition and physical fitness.

OUR STUDY

Twenty obese adolescents, aged 12-15 years with body mass index (BMI) > 25 kg/m2, were recruited via advertisement. Individuals with muscle and bone defects, heart disease, asthma triggered by physical activity, severe illness that requires hospital treatment, taking drugs that affect body composition such as Cushing's syndrome, type I diabetes mellitus, hypothyroid were excluded. Before the baseline tests, the exact details of the study were explained to the participants, screening by a doctor and written informed consent to the study was obtained from each of them and parents. All methods and procedures of the present study were approved by Universitas PGRI Semarang, Indonesia.

Participants were allocated to the FIFA 11+ group. After the baseline test, which measured body composition, physical fitness. The FIFA 11+ group took part in supervised exercise license for 12 weeks. All variables in the baseline tests were measured again at the end of the experiments. The post-intervention tests were performed at least 24 hours after the last training session of FIFA 11+. Under full supervision, all exercise tests and training sessions were conducted in the exercise laboratory of Universitas PGRI Semarang. There were have diet interventions with amount calorie 1700 kcal/day. Physical activity was assessed using an Adolescent Physical Activity Recall Questionnaires (APARQ) (13).

Body mass and height of each participant were measured to calculate their BMI by dividing body mass (kg) by height in meters squared (m2). After an overnight fast, body composition was measured by bioelectrical impedance analysis equipment (Body Composition Analyser Tanita AB-140 Viscan, Tanita Corporation of America, Inc., USA). Height was measured by stadiometer.

VO2max was estimated using the YMCA Cycle Ergometer submaximal test (14). The protocol uses three or more consecutive 3-min workloads that are designed to raise the HR to between 110 bpm and an HR that is near 85% of the age-predicted HRmax for two consecutive workloads. The starting pedalling rate is 50 rpm and the initial workload is 150 kpm.min-1 (25W). The HR during the last minute of the first workload determines the loading sequence of subsequent workloads. For example, if the HR is 80-89 bpm or 90-100 bpm, the respective workloads for the second stage would be 600 or 450 kpm.min-1, respectively. VO2max was then predicted from the estimated maximal HR (220-age) (15). Resting BP was measured by the auscultatory method after 10 minutes of resting.

FIFA 11+ training program

The FIFA 11+ group undertook 12 weeks, one hour per day for three per week. The training session consisted of a 10-minute warm-up period, which included walking and jogging, as well as skeletal muscle stretches. The FIFA 11+ consisted of seven different exercises: a running game, two jumping exercises, a balance/coordination task, two exercises targeting body stability, and an exercise to improve falling technique (table 1). Short breaks of 1-2 minutes were allowed and finally, there was a 10-minutes cool-down period which involved slow walking and skeletal muscle stretches. The researchers supervised all the training sessions.

Table 1. FIFA 11+ training program

Part 1: Running exercise	**8 minutes**
Straight ahead, hip out, hip in circling partner, shoulder contact, quick forwards and backwards	30 m each item 3-5 repetitions 2 sets
Part 2: Strength. Plyometric, Balance	10 minutes
The bench: static	20-30 sec. 2 sets
Sideways bench: static	20-30 sec. 3 sets 10 repetitions on each side
Hamstring beginner	60 sec. 3-5 repetitions 1 set
Single-leg stance: hold the ball	30 s each leg 2 sets
Squats: with toe raise	30 sec. 3-5 repetitions 2 sets
Jumping: vertical jumps	30 sec. 10 jumps 2 sets
Part 3: Running exercise	2 minutes
Across the pitch, bounding, plant and cut	3 running items, 30 m each item 3-5 repetitions 2 sets

Dietary records

All participants recorded a five-weekday dietary diary at the beginning and the end of the experimental period, respectively. The food weight and percentages of carbohydrate, fat, and protein in the food were estimated. Daily energy intake was calculated by multiplying the weight of carbohydrate, fat, and protein consumed by their energy values 1,700 kcal/day. After removing the highest and lowest values, the average of the other three days was reported as the daily energy intake.

Statistical analyses

All analyses were performed using SPSS Version 22 for Windows (SPSS Inc. USA). All values are presented as mean ± SD. The distribution of raw data sets was checked using the Kolmogorov–Smirnov test and demonstrated that all data had a normal distribution ($p < 0.05$).

FINDINGS

The total number of subjects who received the intervention until the end of the program totalled 20 people, two participants dropped out of the study, consisting of 16 men and 4 women, with an average age of 13.6 ± 0.4 years. The mean weight of the subjects was 68.46 ± 10.69 kg. The mean weight of male and female subjects was 70.25 ± 11.13 kg and

Table 2. Results

Subject Characteristics	Total (n = 20)	Men (n = 16)	Women (n = 16)	Pre-test	Post-test	p
Age (years)	13.6 ± 0.4	13.63 ± 0.31	13.29 ± 0.55			
Height (cm)	157.93 ± 6.69	159.53 ± 6.22	151.53 ± 4.65			
Weight (kg)	68.46 ± 10.69	70.25 ± 11.13	61.3 ± 4.41			
BMI (kg/m^2)	27.36 ± 2.09	27.52 ± 3.48	26.72 ± 1.95	27.36 ± 2.09	26.84 ± 3.42	0.02*
VO_2max (ml/kg/min)	25.6 ± 3.3	25.8 ± 3.39	24.75 ± 2.70	25.6 ± 3.3	30.15 ± 9.58	0.029*
Energi intake (kcal/day)	2455.55 ± 417.88	2479.5 ± 398.92	2359.75 ± 543.11	2455.55 ± 417.88	2163 ± 401.22	0.008*

*t-test.

61.3 ± 4.41 kg. The mean height of the subjects was 157.93 ± 6.69 cm. The mean height of male and female subjects was 159.52 ± 6.22 cm and 151.53 ± 4.65 cm.

The mean BMI of the subjects was 27.36 ± 2,095 kg/m2. The mean BMI of male and female subjects was 27.52 ± 3.47 kg/m2 and 26.72 ± 1.95 kg/m2. The mean VO2max prediction based on the results of the YMCA cycle ergometer submaximal is 25.6 ± 3.3 ml/kg/min. The mean VO2max for male subjects was 25.8 ± 3.4 ml/kg/min, whereas for female subjects it was 24.75 ± 2.7 ml/kg/min.

The mean calorie intake of subjects before the intervention was 2455.55 ± 417.88 kcal/day. The mean caloric intake in men is 2479.5 ±

398.9 kcal/day and 2359.75 ± 543.1 kcal/day (Table 2). The level of daily physical activity of the subjects is mostly included in the inactive category, while others are included in the vigorous category.

Discussion

All subjects belong to the adolescent category where this period is a period of rapid growth and there is a dramatic change in body composition influenced by physical activity and response to exercise. There is an increase in bone size and muscle mass and there is a change in the size and distribution of fat storage body (16). This is the reason for selecting the age group in this study. In this study, the mean BMI in subjects dropped significantly (p = 0.02) after intervention. In male subjects, the mean of BMI was significantly decreased (p = 0.022), whereas, in female subjects, there was a decrease in BMI that was not statistically significant (p = 0.38). Changes in BMI in female subjects cannot be analyzed properly due to the limited number of subjects. Weight loss in the subjects allegedly caused by a reduction in the percentage of body fat mass with varying amounts. This is consistent with a meta-analysis of research with exercise as a method for the management of obesity. Obtained a decrease in body fat percent that is monitored after an exercise program, with the factors estimated as the main predictors are the duration (minutes) of exercise, the amount of time the exercise program, and a combination of types of exercise (aerobic exercise and endurance) (17).

The cardiorespiratory fitness level of subjects before intervention on the subject is very far below the average obtained based on research Quinart et al. (18) showing a VO2max value of 54.9 ± 8.4 ml/kg/min in men and 47.4 ± 6.2 ml/kg/min in women. The level of physical fitness of subjects before and after the intervention found a significant difference (p = 0.029) between the YMCA cycle ergometer submaximal test before and after the intervention. Increased levels of cardiovascular freshness are caused due to the adaptation of the heart and lungs to exercise. In the cardiovascular system there is an increase in cardiac output which aims to maintain the skeletal muscles that are at work so that there is an increase in blood flow to meet the needs of oxygen and nutrients for muscle cells and carry carbon monoxide and metabolic waste to the disposal site (19–21). An increase in cardiac output is thought to be due to sympathetic stimulation which increases heart rate and strength of heart muscle contraction, and reduced parasympathetic excitement to the heart; vascular vasodilation in skeletal muscles; respiratory activation which increases venous return and peripheral vasodilation thereby increasing stroke volume. Adaptation to the respiratory system, an increase in blood flow through the pulmonary capillaries (increased lung perfusion), an increase in the frequency and depth of breathing (ventilation) and an increase in the rate of diffusion of oxygen from the lungs to the blood and carbon dioxide from the blood to the lungs (19–21).

Research conducted Watts et al (19) of obese adolescents who were given circuit training interventions by doing exercises using bicycle ergometers and endurance training for 8 weeks, with frequency of exercise three times a week and duration of 1 hour that has been proven to improve functional capacity, muscle endurance, and body composition, and furthermore, can improve blood fat profile. The study Gutin et al (22) also reported similar results where the level of cardiovascular freshness in adolescent obese increased significantly with physical exercise. In this study also reported exercise also reduces levels of visceral fat and total body fat, but it is not clear about the effects of the intensity of physical exercise. An increase in the level of cardiorespiratory freshness occurred in male subjects significantly ($p = 0.029$), but the opposite results were shown in female subjects where there was a significant decrease in the level of cardio respiration freshness ($p = 0.477$). This might be due to observations during the intervention on a limited number of female subjects, lack of motivation in female subjects and a feeling of being reluctant to practice if their friends were not present so the exercise program could not be effectively carried out.

Nutrition education and dietary information carried out simultaneously with exercise interventions on subjects succeeded in changing the subject's diet, as evidenced by a significant reduction in calorie intake ($p = 0.008$). This is a confounding factor that influences the results of this study. The goal of decreasing 1,700 kcal/day cannot be fulfilled because researchers cannot supervise and provide full intervention as was done on quarantined subjects. Subjects still determine the diet to be consumed while at home and also determined by the family's diet. The effect of changes in calorie intake is greater than the effect of exercise interventions on changes in BMI. These results are in line with research Deforche et al. (23) on women and men that increased calorie intake is the biggest predictor of improvement in BMI, compared to TV/game/video viewing time, and lack of physical activity. Research Ben Ounis et al. (24) states that a comparison between dietary intake restriction programs and dietary intake restriction exercise shows better changes in body weight and fitness levels in sports groups with dietary intake restrictions. A 4-month intervention with 250 kcal exercise per session with a low-calorie intake showed a greater change in BMI compared to intervention with only a low-calorie intake.

The limitation of this study is the lack of female subjects at the time of the intervention resulted in an analysis of the results of the intervention could not be optimal. The number of obesity students who are not willing to take part in research is due to the tight school schedule and reluctance to take part in sports.

Conclusion

Obese adolescents and the whole family need to be given an understanding that diet and exercise are not completed when weight loss can be achieved, but calorie restriction must be carried out and become a daily habit. Exercise programs and dietary arrangements are sought to be specifically included in school health programs as part of school health efforts, under the supervision of a doctor.

ACKNOWLEDGEMENTS

The research was funded by the Khon Kaen University. The author thanks the research investigator and study participants. The authors declare that there is no conflict of interest.

REFERENCES

[1] Ng M, Fleming T, Robinson M, Thomson B, Graetz N, Margono C, et al. Global, regional, and national prevalence of overweight and obesity in children and adults during 1980-2013: a systematic analysis for the global burden of disease study 2013. Lancet 2014;384(9945):766-81.

[2] Kesehatan K, Indonesia R, Ibu K, Anak K, Menular P, Tidak P, et al. Potret sehat Indonesia dari riskesdas 2018. Indonesia: Ministry of Health Republic of Indonesia, 2019. [Indonesian]

[3] Centers for disease control and prevention: adult obesity facts. NCHS Data Brief 2017;288:1-8.

[4] Donnelly JE, Blair SN, Jakicic JM, Manore MM, Rankin JW, Smith BK. Appropriate physical activity intervention strategies for weight loss and prevention of weight regain for adults. Med Sci Sports Exerc 2009;41(2):459-71.

[5] Crichton GE, Alkerwi A. Physical activity, sedentary behavior time and lipid levels in the observation of cardiovascular risk factors in Luxembourg study. Lipids Health Dis 2015;14:87.

[6] Fisher G, Brown AW, Bohan Brown MM, Alcorn A, Noles C, Winwood L, et al. High intensity interval vs moderate intensity-training for improving cardiometabolic health in overweight or obese males: a randomized controlled trial. PloS One 2015;10(10):e0138853.

[7] Christ M, Iannello C, Iannello PG, Grimm W. Effects of a weight reduction program with and without aerobic exercise in the metabolic syndrome. Int J Cardiol 2004;97(1):115-22.

[8] Ryan AS, Nicklas BJ, Berman DM. Aerobic exercise is necessary to improve glucose utilization with moderate weight loss in women. Obesity (Silver Spring) 2006;14(6):1064-72.

[9] Slentz CA, Duscha BD, Johnson JL. Effects of the amount of exercise on body weight, body composition and measures of central obesity. Arch Intern Med 2004;164(1):31-9.

[10] Fuller CW, Ørntoft C, Larsen MN, Elbe AM, Ottesen L, Junge A, et al. "FIFA 11 for Health" for Europe 1: effect on health knowledge and well-being of 10 to 12-year-old Danish school children. Br J Sports Med 2017;51(20):1483-8.

[11] Tan S, Wang X, Wang J. Effects of supervised exercise training at the intensity of maximal fat oxidation in overweight young women. J Exerc Sci Fit 2012;10(2);64-9.

[12] Lanzi S, Codecasa F, Cornacchia M, Maestrini S, Capodaglio P, Brunani A, et al. Short-term HIIT and fat training increase aerobic and metabolic fitness in men with class II and III obesity. Obesity (Silver Spring) 2015;23(10):1987-94.

[13] Booth ML, Okely AD, Chey T, Bauman A. The reliability and validity of the adolescent physical activity recall questionnaire. Med Sci Sports Exerc 2002;34(12):1986-95.

[14] Golding L, Sinning W. Y's Way to Physical Fitness: the complete guide to fitness testing and instruction: YMCA of the USA. Champaign, IL: Human Kinetics Publishers, 1989.

[15] Linda S Pescatello; American College of Sports Medicine. ACSM's guidelines for exercise testing and prescription 9th ed. 2014. Philadelphia, PA: Wolters Kluwer/Lippincott Williams Wilkins Health, 2014.

[16] Salam RA, Hooda M, Das JK, Arshad A, Lassi ZS, Middleton P, et al. Interventions to improve adolescent nutrition: a systematic review and meta-Analysis. J Adolesc Health 2016;59(4S):S29-S39.

[17] Maziekas MT, LeMura LM, Stoddard NM, Kaercher S, Martucci T. Follow up exercise studies in paediatric obesity: implications for long term effectiveness. Br J Sports Med 2003;37(5):425-9.

[18] Quinart S, Mougin F, Simon-Rigaud ML, Nicolet-Guénat M, Nègre V, Regnard J. Evaluation of cardiorespiratory fitness using three field tests in obese adolescents: validity, sensitivity and prediction of peak V̇O2. J Sci Med Sport 2014;17(5):521-5.

[19] Watts K, Jones TW, Davis EA, Green D. Exercise training in obese children and adolescents: current concepts. Sports Med 2005;35(5):375-92.

[20] Watts K, Beye P, Siafarikas A, Davis EA, Jones TW, Driscoll G, et al. Exercise training normalizes vascular dysfunction and improves central adiposity in obese adolescents. J Am Coll Cardiol 2004;43(10):1823-7.

[21] Mendelson M, Michallet AS, Estève F, Perrin C, Levy P, Wuyam B, et al. Ventilatory responses to exercise training in obese adolescents. Respir Physiol Neurobiol 2012;184(1):73-9.

[22] Gutin B, Barbeau P, Owens S, Lemmon CR, Bauman M, Allison J, et al. Effects of exercise intensity on cardiovascular fitness total body composition and visceral adiposity of obese adolescents. Am J Clin Nutr 2002;75(5):818-26.

[23] Deforche B, Van Dyck D, Deliens T, De Bourdeaudhuij I. Changes in weight physical activity sedentary behaviour and dietary intake during the transition to higher education: a prospective study. Int J Behav Nutr Phys Act 2015;12:16.

[24] Ben Ounis O, Elloumi M, Amri M, Trabelsi Y, Lac G, Tabka Z. Impact of training and hypocaloric diet on fat oxidation and body composition in obese adolescents. Sci Sports 2009;24(3–4):178–85.

In: Pediatrics and Adolescent Health ISBN: 978-1-68507-490-6
Editors: J. Merrick and M. Morad

Chapter 4

CARE PATHWAYS AND OUT OF POCKET EXPENDITURE AMONG CHILDREN WITH TUBERCULOSIS ATTENDING A TERTIARY HEALTH CARE FACILITY

Kamya Rangarajan[1], Jeby Jose Olickal[1], Revathi Ulaganeethi[1], Palanivel Chinnakali[1,*], MD, Shanthosh Priyan Sundaram[1], MD and Niranjan Biswal[2], MD

[1]Department of Preventive and Social Medicine, Jawaharlal Institute of Postgraduate Medicine and Research (JIPMER), Puducherry, India
[2]Department of Pediatrics, Jawaharlal Institute of Postgraduate Medicine and Research (JIPMER), Puducherry, India

[*] Corresponding Author's E-mail: palaniccm@gmail.com.

ABSTRACT

In this chapter we aim to describe the providers and out of pocket expenditure involved in the care of childhood tuberculosis (TB). Methods: We conducted a facility based descriptive study at a pediatric outpatient clinic between March and July 2018. Information on symptoms, number and sequence of providers and the expenditure were captured through interviews with parents. Results: A total of 73 children were included, mean age was 9.8 years and more than half were females (57.5%). Most (57.5%) reported fever as the first symptom. Regarding first point of contact, 57% sought care at public health facilities, 40% at private hospital or clinic and two (3%) children were taken to a traditional healer. Median (range) of providers visited in the entire pathways of TB care was one (1-2). Median (IQR) time gap between first symptom and diagnosis was 30 (0-30) days in children who contacted private provider or traditional healer. Financial constraints were the major reason for the preference of the first point of contact and the median (IQR) money spent on the entire pathways was 37.1 (23-54.9) USD. Conclusion: More than half of children diagnosed with TB had sought care at public health facilities and there was a substantial delay in diagnosis among children seeking care from private providers and traditional healer.

INTRODUCTION

According to the World Health Organization (WHO), tuberculosis (TB) is one of the top ten causes of death and the leading cause from a single infectious agent. In 2018, globally the estimated incidence of TB cases was 10 million, of which 1.0 million (10%) was among children (1). TB is a major cause of deaths in children, despite not being recorded as such, and is likely in the top ten causes of global mortality in this age group (2–5). The actual burden of TB in children is likely to be higher given the challenge in diagnosing childhood TB. The increased incidence of TB in children shows the continuing transmission within a community (6) and United Nations in its sustainable development goals have committed to end preventable deaths in children by 2030. Addressing the delays in diagnosis and early initiation on anti-tuberculosis therapy is vital to achieve this goal. Fear of stigma and isolation from peer group adds as a burden for the children with TB (1).

In India, the majority of the children with TB predominantly seek care and more than 50% are diagnosed and treated in private hospitals. The majority of the private sectors are individual providers, who are both formal (qualified) and informal (nonqualified) providers. The Stop TB Partnership's global plan to end TB 2016-2020 estimates that in developing countries 10.4 billion US dollar was needed in 2018 increasing to US$12.3 billion in 2020 for the prevention, diagnosis, and treatment of TB(1). It shows the need to study the out of pocket expenditure incurred by individual for the care of TB. There are only a limited number of studies from India capturing the pathways and costs related to children with TB. In the current study, we aim to assess the pathways of care for children with TB, who were diagnosed at a tertiary care hospital in South India and to provide an estimate of the cost spent on pathways during the diagnosis of TB.

OUR STUDY

This facility-based descriptive study was conducted among the children diagnosed with TB registering at the pediatric outpatient clinic of a tertiary care hospital, Puducherry, South India during March to July 2018. Children diagnosed with multi-drug resistant TB were excluded.

Information on the number of providers, the provider of the first contact, the duration between providers, direct costs including medication charges, doctor consultation fee, laboratory expenses and indirect costs including transport charges, loss of wages of the parent/ caretaker were assessed using a semi-structured questionnaire from parents/caretaker. Disease related information was extracted from medical records.

Table 1. Distribution of Socio-demographic characteristics of the children diagnosed with TB at a tertiary care center, Puducherry, 2018 (N=73)

Variable	N	%
Age in years		
<5	23	31.5
6-10	15	20.6
11-15	19	26
>15	16	21.9
Gender		
Male	31	42.5
Female	42	57.5
Residence		
Rural	31	42.5
Urban	42	57.5
Fathers Occupation		
Daily Waged	47	64.4
Monthly Waged	17	23.3
Farmer	8	11
Unemployed	1	1.4
Education		
No formal education	12	16.4
1-8	30	41.1
9-10	24	32.9
11-12	7	9.6
Socio-economic class*		
Class 1 (6574 and above)	1	1.4
Class 2 (3287-6573)	10	13.9
Class 3 (1972-3286)	18	25
Class 4 (986-1971)	38	52.8
Class 5 (985 and below)	10	13.9

*Updated BG Prasad's social classification as per May 2018.

Data was entered in EpiCollect5 (mobile application) and analysis was done using Stata version 14. Continuous variables like age and family income were summarized as mean (standard deviation) and median (interquartile range). Categorical variables like father's occupation, education status, socio-economic status, and place residence were summarized as proportion. Pathways to care were depicted as a flow diagram using number of children seeking care at each level. The direct and indirect costs incurred from the onset of symptoms until diagnosis were summarized as median (IQR) and the costs were converted to US dollars (conversion rate as on May 2018).

The study protocol was reviewed and approved by the institutional ethics committee. Written informed consent was obtained from the parents/caretaker at the time of recruitment after explaining the purpose of the study. For children between 7 and 12 years, verbal/oral assent was obtained in the presence of the parents/caretaker and was recorded. For children between 12 and 18 years, written assent was obtained. Confidentiality and privacy were maintained during the interview.

OUR FINDINGS

A total of 73 children diagnosed with TB were included. The mean (SD) age of children was 9.8 (5) years. Distribution of socio-demographic characteristics (see Table 1) showed that the majority of the children were in the age group of less than five years (31.5%) and more than half were females (57.5%). More than half of the children (57.5%) reported first symptom as fever and cough followed by body/abdominal pain (32.9%) (see Table 2).

Pathways undertaken to seek care (Flowchart 1) shows that 42 (57.5%) children approached a public health facility as their first point of care where the DOTS was provided. Of the rest, 29 (39.7%) of them went to a private clinic (Non-DOTS) and 2 (2.7%) went to traditional healer. Out of those two children who went to a traditional healer, one went to a general hospital and another one to a private hospital as their second point of care.

Reasons for preference for the first point of contact (see Table 3) showed that the majority of the people (60%) who had financial constraints approached a public tertiary care hospital followed by the general hospital (40%). Faith was considered a reason for preference only by the people who approached traditional healer (100%). Distance was given as a reason by a majority of the people who approached a private hospital/clinic (49%). Relatives were the decision makers in 70% of the cases followed by parents (22%). Median (IQR) time gap between first symptom and TB diagnosis was 30 (0-30) days in children who contacted Private provider or traditional healer.

Table 2. Distribution of first symptoms developed, the first point of contact and the decision maker for the first point of contact among children diagnosed with TB at a tertiary care center, Puducherry, 2018 (N=73)

Variable	N	%
First symptoms developed		
Fever and cough	42	57.5
Body/Abdominal Pain	24	32.9
Seizure	4	5.5
Lesions	2	2.7
Swelling	1	1.4
First point of contact		
Native/religious healer	2	2.7
General Hospital (DOTS Center)	25	34.3
Tertiary Care Hospital (DOTS Center)	17	23.3
PVT/ Govt. Hospitals/Clinics (Non-DOTS)	29	39.7
Decision maker for the first point of contact		
Relatives	54	74
Parents	16	21.9
Neighbours	2	2.7
Patient him/herself	1	1.4

Total median (IQR) cost during the pathways to TB care was 37.1 (23- 54.9) USD; median (IQR) direct cost was 1.5 (0-4.4) USD and median indirect (IQR) cost was 32.2 (22.2- 52.6) USD. The direct and indirect cost incurred from the onset of symptoms till reaching DOTS (see Table 5) showed that, direct cost was none if the diagnosis was made at public health facility but indirect cost accounted for 16.7 USD on an average with an IQR 9.7-29.7 USD.

Table 3. Reason for preference for the first point of contact among children diagnosed with TB at a tertiary care center, Puducherry, 2018 (N=73)

Reasons for preference	Native/religious healer (n=2)	General hospital (n=25)	Tertiary care hospital (n=17)	Private hospitals/clinics [Non-DOTS] (n=29)
	n (%)	n (%)	n (%)	n (%)
Financial reasons	0	6 (40)	9 (60)	0
Faith	1 (100)	0	0	0
Distance	0	17 (41.5)	4 (9.8)	20 (48.8)
Close relative reference	1 (7.1)	2 (14.3)	3 (21.4)	8 (57.1)
Other reasons*	0	0	0	2 (100)

*good quality+ no specific reason.

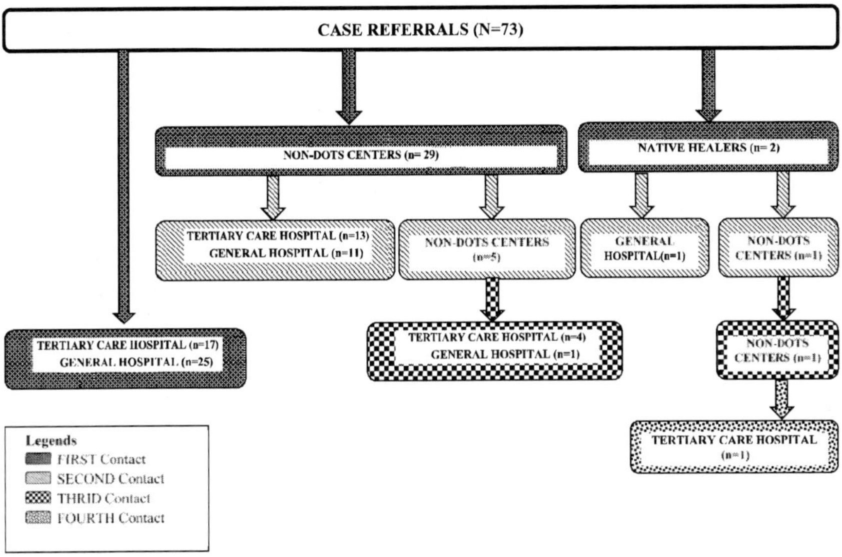

Figure 1. Pathways undertaken to seek care by children diagnosed with TB at a tertiary care Centre, Puducherry, 2018.

Table 4. Decision maker for the first point of care among children diagnosed with TB at a tertiary care center, Puducherry, 2018 (N=73)

First Contact	Patient him/herself n (%)	Relative n (%)	Neighbours n (%)	Parents n (%)
Native/religious healer (2)	0	1 (50)	1 (50)	0
General hospital (25)	0	18 (72)	0	7 (28)
Tertiary care hospital (17)	0	12 (70.6)	0	5 (29.4)
Private hospitals/ clinics (29)	1 (3.5)	23 (74)	1 (3.5)	4 (13.8)

Table 5. The direct and indirect cost incurred from the onset of symptoms until reaching DOTS among children diagnosed with TB at a tertiary care center, Puducherry, 2018 (N=73)

Diagnosis at	N (%)	Median (IQR) Cost (in USD)		
		Direct*	Indirect†	Total‡
1st point of contact	42	0 (0-0)	16.7 (9.7-29.7)	17.1 (9.7-31.2)
2nd point of contact	25	2.2 (1.5-40.6)	23.7 (14.1-23.7)	27.2 (17.2-40.6)
3rd point of contact	5	8.2 (4.6-18.3)	46.9 (26.7-78.2)	60.6 (35.6-87.1)
4th point of contact	1	22.2 (22.2-22.2)	71.8(71.8-71.8)	94.0 (94.0-94.0)

*Consultation fee + Medicine charges + Laboratory charges.

†Patient food charges + Caretaker food charges + Patient transportation charges + Caretaker transportation charges + Patient loss of wages + caretakers loss of wages + Patient other expenses + Caretakers Other expenses.

‡ Direct cost + Indirect cost

The median (IQR) cost for total pathways of TB care was 46 (25.2-68.2) USD for those who went to private provider or traditional healers for their first contact compared to 30 (25.2-48.2) USD for those who approached public health facilities. Direct and indirect cost increased with the increase in the number of providers or the diagnosis of TB was farther in the cascade.

DISCUSSION

Our study found that about two fifths of the pediatric TB cases reported to non-RNTCP facilities as first contact. A similar study by Kapoor et al. (7) on adult TB patients in Delhi reported that informal providers and retail chemist were the first point of contact for two third of patients. The current study reported that the decision maker for the first point of contact among 74% of the participants were relatives or family members because relatives act as the major decision-makers during illness. In our study, one participant approached DOTS facility in his/her fourth contact for care and eight children approached in their third point of contact for care and the other studies (7–9) also reported similar findings.

Among those who contacted private provider, availability close to their residence was reported as a reason for preference. Faith and family reference were the reason for approaching traditional healer for paediatric TB care. A study from Delhi reported a similar finding for patients with mental health problems for availing care from non- specialists (10).

The time gap between onset of symptoms and diagnosis was about a month in children who visited the private providers or traditional healer. Considering the infectious nature of TB, earlier diagnosis would have reduced transmission of the disease and morbidity. However, in the absence of cough/fever, symptoms in the childhood TB can be non-specific and can explain the delay in such cases. Raising awareness in general population and grass root level health care workers about the possibility of TB in children with undernutrition will help in early diagnosis of TB in the community. Also, strengthening the public-private mix model in TB care by involving private providers will improve TB case detection and notification.

Our study found that total cost was higher in private sector compared to public health facilities. These findings are similar to the studies conducted by Sandra et al. (11) and Kemp et al. (12). A community-based mental health study was conducted by Amaddeo et al. (13) on accessibility and pathways to psychiatric care in a community also reported the similar trends in out of pocket expenditure.

The study had limitations. Our study participants were from a tertiary care center with additional facilities for TB diagnosis especially extra-pulmonary tuberculosis and hence findings may not be generalizable to other settings. Possibility of recall limitation cannot be ruled out especially with the expenditure spent during the pathways. To the best of our knowledge this is the first study describing the pathways to care in childhood TB in India.

Conclusion

Two fifths children diagnosed with TB had their first contact at a non-DOTS center and had a substantial delay from onset of symptoms to TB diagnosis and initiation of treatment. More sustained efforts are needed to sensitize the private providers and traditional healers to improve TB case detection and notification.

Conflict of Interest

No conflict of interest declared.

References

[1] World Health Organization. Global tuberculosis report 2018. Geneva: World Health Organization, 2018.

[2] Dodd PJ, Gardiner E, Coghlan R, Seddon JA. Burden of childhood tuberculosis in 22 high-burden countries: A mathematical modelling study. Lancet Glob Health 2014;2(8):453–9.

[3] Graham SM, Sismanidis C, Menzies HJ, Marais BJ, Detjen AK, Black RE. Importance of tuberculosis control to address child survival. Lancet 2014;383(9928):1605–7.

[4] Marais BJ, Graham SM, Maeurer M, Zumla A. Progress and challenges in childhood tuberculosis. Lancet Infect Dis 2013;13(4):287–9.

[5] Jenkins HE. Global burden of childhood tuberculosis. Pneumonia 2016;8(1):24–30.

[6] World Health Organization. Roadmap for childhood tuberculosis: Towards zero deaths. Geneva: World Health Organization, 2013.

[7] Kapoor SK, Raman AV, Sachdeva KS, Satyanarayana S. How did the TB patients reach DOTS services in Delhi? A study of patient treatment seeking behavior. PLoS One 2012;7:8.

[8] Joshi B, Chinnakali P, Shrestha A, Das M, Kumar AMV, Pant R, et al. Impact of intensified case-finding strategies on childhood TB case registration in Nepal. Public Health Action 2015;5(2):93–8.

[9] Chadda R, Mishra N, Nagpal S, Sood M. Help-seeking behavior of patients with mental health problems visiting a tertiary care center in North India. Indian J Psychiatry 2011;53(3):234–9.

[10] Lahariya C, Singhal S, Gupta S, Mishra A. Pathway of care among psychiatric patients attending a mental health institution in central India. Indian J Psychiatry 2010;52(4):333–8.

[11] Kik S V, Olthof SP, de Vries JT, Menzies D, Kincler N, van Loenhout-Rooyakkers J, et al. Direct and indirect costs of tuberculosis among immigrant patients in the Netherlands. BMC Public Health 2009;9(1):283–91.

[12] Kemp JR, Mann G, Simwaka BN, Salaniponi FM, Squire SB. Can Malawi's poor afford free tuberculosis services? Patient and household costs associated with a tuberculosis diagnosis in Lilongwe. Bull World Health Organ 2007;85:580–5.

[13] Amaddeo F, Zambello F, Tansella M, Thornicroft G. Accessibility and pathways to psychiatric care in a community-based mental health system. Soc Psychiatry Psychiatr Epidemiol 2001;36(10):500–7.

In: Pediatrics and Adolescent Health ISBN: 978-1-68507-490-6
Editors: J. Merrick and M. Morad

Chapter 5

UNDERNUTRITION AND ITS DETERMINANTS AMONG INDIGENOUS THAMI CHILDREN UNDER FIVE IN THE DOLAKHA DISTRICT OF NEPAL

Keshav Dahal and Montakarn Chuemchit**, PhD
College of Public Health Sciences and Health and Social Sciences
and Addiction Research Unit, Chulalongkorn University,
Patumwan, Bangkok, Thailand

ABSTRACT

Stunting, wasting, and being underweight are major public health issues leading to morbidity and mortality in under-five children. The prevalence of these issues is especially high in low-income countries with socially deprived and marginalized population groups. This study aimed to determine the prevalence of undernutrition and its determinants among under-five children of indigenous Thami population in the Dolakha district of Nepal. Methods: A community-

* Corresponding Author's E-mail: montakarn.ch@chula.ac.th.

based quantitative cross-sectional study was conducted with a multistage sampling of 366 under-five children and their biological mothers. Anthropometric data were collected as per WHO guidelines, and WHO Anthro software was used to assess the prevalence of stunting, wasting, and being underweight. SPSS was used for descriptive statistics and chi-square tests. Results: Among the surveyed children, 8.5% experienced wasting, 43.7% experienced stunting, and 27.6% were underweight. Higher prevalence rates for all three forms of undernutrition occurred in the age group of 11–23 months. The number of children in a family using the same cooking pot, the mother's age at last delivery, contraceptive use, and introduction of other food items to children immediately after birth were significantly associated with stunting. Similarly, the mothers' occupations, postnatal check-ups, vitamin A intake during the postpartum period, use of contraceptives, and consumption of alcohol during pregnancy were significantly associated with being underweight. Conclusion: Undernutrition is still an alarming issue with a high prevalence among under-five children. Intervention in health risk behaviors and health service utilization may reduce childhood undernutrition.

Keyword: prevalence, undernutrition, under-five children, indigenous, Nepal

INTRODUCTION

Undernutrition includes being underweight, wasting, stunting, and having micronutrient deficiencies or insufficiencies. Undernutrition is a serious, long-lasting, and challenging problem for individuals, families, communities, and countries. Undernutrition affects medical and socioeconomic development (1, 2), including morbidity and mortality. Approximately 3.1 million (45%) deaths of under-five children are due to undernutrition, mostly in low and middle-income countries (3). In 2016, pneumonia, diarrhea, and malaria were leading causes of under-five deaths, occurring in approximately 16% and 8% under-five children. Mortality of under-five children is strongly associated with undernutrition, lack of sanitation and safe water, and poor access to health care (1).

Globally, in 2017, 22% of children experienced stunting, 7.5% experienced wasting, and 5.6% were undernourished (4). Two out of five children experience stunting in southern Asia, and more than half of children under five experience wasting (3). Undernutrition causes growth failure, resulting in underweight and stunted children with poor physical and emotional states and less intellectual productivity (5). Children with disabilities are almost three times more likely to be underweight and nearly twice as likely to experience stunting, wasting, neurodevelopmental disability, and hearing impairments (6).

Undernutrition can reduce children's immunological function, leading to inadequate responses to infectious agents (7). Undernourished children suffer from frequent infections with high severity and succumb more often to infectious illnesses. Response to infectious illnesses is a major determinant of the standard of living, quality of life, and, ultimately, overall social and economic development. Low-income family, lower maternal education, poor water supply, nonaccess to health services, large family size, incomplete vaccinations, poor household sanitation, low birth orders, frequent illness, poor maternal health nutrition, and inappropriate infant and young child feeding and care in early life are associated with all three forms of undernutrition (8).

Nepal still has very high prevalences of stunting and wasting (>30% and >15%, respectively) in children under the age of five. According to the National Demographic and Health Survey (NDHS) of 2016, the prevalence of stunting, wasting, and underweight among under-five children was 36%, 10%, and 27%, respectively. Stunting is more common in rural children (40%) than in urban children. Even though many international and national nonprofit organizations work with the Ministry of Health and the nutrition sector, no satisfactory decrease in undernutrition has occurred relative to the millennium development goals and sustainable development goals for nutrition.

Among 62 indigenous ethnic population groups, 91.3% of the indigenous Thami population resides in rural areas of Nepal (9). The magnitude of undernutrition and its determinants among under-five children from the indigenous ethnic groups of Thami from Nepal are poorly understood. Due to the high prevalence and consequences, undernutrition is still a global challenge, especially in middle-lower- and lower-income countries. This study was conducted to determine the prevalence of undernutrition and its determinants among indigenous Nepalese Thami children under five. Data concerning socioeconomic characteristics, mother-related factors, and child-related factors were collected under the WHO guidelines for anthropometric measurements and definitions and classification of undernutrition.

METHODS

A community-based quantitative cross-sectional study was conducted among children under five from the indigenous Thami population in the Dolakha district of Nepal from 18 August 2019 to 25 September 2019. The Dolakha district is the ancestral land of the indigenous Thami population. According to the National Population and Household Survey (NPHS) of 2011, the total number of indigenous Thami was 28,671, which is 0.1% of the national population, and 16,597 (57.9%) of the Thami resided only in the Dolakha district, accounting for 8.9% of the total population of that district.

Approximately 75% of the indigenous Thami population resided in the central mountain region of the country. The growth rate was 2.2, average household size was 4.5, sex ratio was 94% (male:female), male dependency ratio was 85%, and female dependency ratio was 76.9%. Approximately 75% of the population was involved in traditional farming. Only 5.5% of households used clean cooking energy. Approximately 80% of households used improved drinking water sources, and 64.5% of households had toilet facilities. The female literacy rate was 50.5%, and male literacy rate was 57.4% (10).

Sampling and sample size

The study population included mothers and their children under five years of age from the Thami indigenous population. The current indigenous Thami population of Dolakha district was calculated by applying Pt = P(1+r/100)t with an indigenous Thami population growth rate of 2.20, based on the NPHS of 2011. The total population of the under-five indigenous Thami population was projected to be 7.36% from the hilly district, according to the NPHS of 2011.

The sample size was calculated from the projected population. The projected final population of Thami ethnicity was calculated as 19,753, and the number of under-five children was projected to be 1,454 by 2019. The Thami population resides only in 24 VDC of the Dolakha district (10). The national prevalence of being underweight was 27% (NDHS-2016), with a 95% confidence interval (CI) and allowable or marginal error (L) of 5%. A nonresponse rate of 10% was considered when calculating the required sample size, which was calculated as n = 366. The required sample size (366) was calculated using the reference value of underweight (27%) with a 95% CI.

A multistage sampling technique was applied to select the district and villages. The Dolakha district was selected using a purposive method, and the sampling frame included eight villages (Lapilang, Melung, Suspa-chhemawoti, Marbu, Sundrawoti, Lakuridada, Kalinchowk, and Dadakharka) using simple random sampling. Sample sizes were calculated for each village using a proportionate sampling technique to reduce selection bias. Four villages (Kalinchowk-ward no. 1, Lapilang-ward no. 5 and 6, Sundrawoti-9 of the Kalinchowk rural municipality, and Chhemawoti-ward no. 1 of the Bhimeshwor municipality) were selected purposively from eight villages, where more than 30 under-five children were residing. The simple random sampling technique was then carried out in each village with the help of the local health institution's vitamin A supplementation and immunization registries.

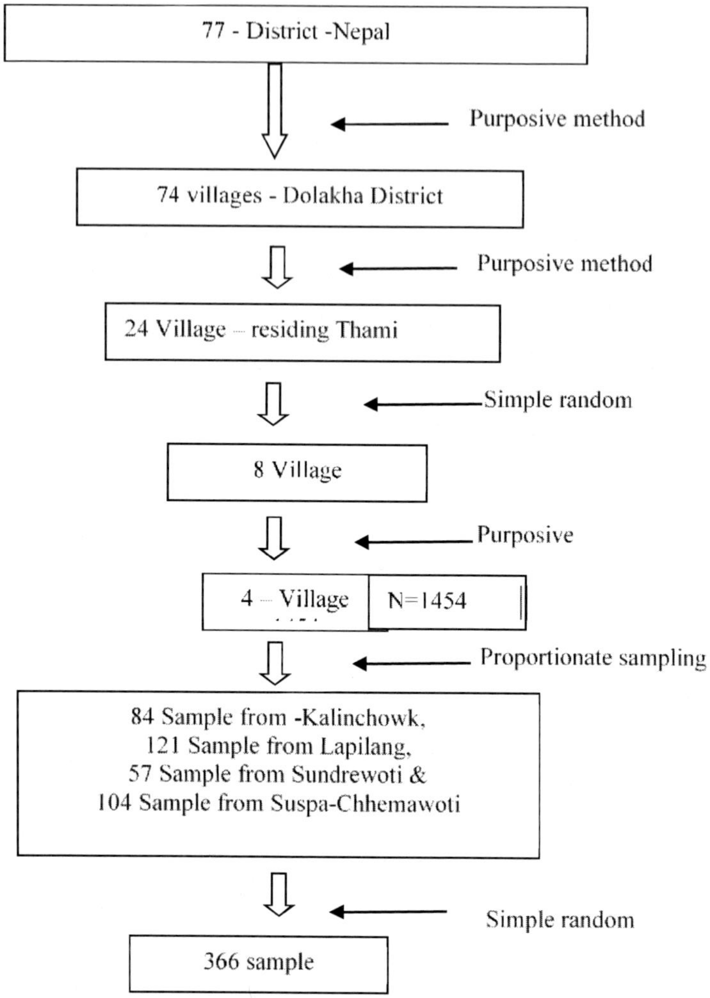

Figure 1. Consort chart.

The questionnaires were prepared according to the NPHS of 2011 and NDHS of 2016 to survey sociodemographic factors, mother-related factors, child-related factors, weights and heights of mothers, and weights and heights/lengths of children residing in the study area for at least 6 months. Questionnaires were restructured and modified according to the existing national level and WHO guidelines for nutrition, family planning, and immunization. The modifications made the questionnaire more suitable to the current study of undernutrition and its determinants. Item-objective congruence was carried out by one nutrition expert and two examiner committee members. A subject expert evaluated English and Nepali languages before implementing the questionnaire. Chulalongkorn University gave ethical approval.

Face-to-face interviews were performed with the mother of under-five children using a semistructured questionnaire and anthropometric measurement tools. Informed consent from the individual respondents was obtained before the interview process and anthropometric measurements of the child. A digital weight machine (Seca model number 876) was used to measure children's and mothers' weights. The weights of the mothers were measured in the standing position. The weights of children aged <2 years were measured with the mother holding the baby after zeroing the mother's weight. The weights of children aged ≥2 years were measured in the standing position. Lengths were measured in the recumbent position for children aged <2 years, and heights were measured in the standing position for children aged ≥2 years. No physically disabled children participated in the study. The exclusion criteria included pregnancy, mothers outside the study area, and temporary residents who have lived in the study area for <6 months. The principal researcher trained the research assistant for interviewing and collecting anthropometric measurements.

Data entry and analysis

The questionnaire was checked and coded before entering data. Data were processed using SPSS software version 22 (licensed from Chulalongkorn University) for Windows. Most sociodemographic, maternal, and child-related determinants were categorical variables and the anthropometric measurements were continuous variables. Descriptive statistics were applied to calculate frequency, percentage, mean, median, and standard deviation. The prevalences of undernutrition (wasting:

weight for height/length; stunting: height for age; and underweight: weight for age) were calculated using WHO Anthro software (version 3.3.2, January 2011) with the WHO reference values for Z-scores. A Chi-square test was applied to identify the association between determinants and undernutrition.

RESULTS

Among 366 children under the age of five, 31 children (8.5%) experienced wasting (weight for height), 160 children (43.7%) experienced stunting (height for age), and 101 children (27.6%) were underweight (weight for age). Growth was severely stunted in 29.5% of children, 6% were severely underweight, and 21.6% were moderately underweight. The highest rate of wasting (< −2 SD; nearly half of the total wasting children) occurred between 12 and 23 months. A higher prevalence of low weight for length/height occurred in children between the ages of 12–23 months, and a higher prevalence of low weight for age occurred in children between the ages of 24–35 months in both the sexes.

Sociodemographic factors

Table 1 shows the study population's sociodemographic factors.

The highest percentage of under-five children was between the ages of 12 and 23 months (29.8%), followed by 12–23 months (19.4%), 24–35 months (19.4%), 36–47 months (12.6%), and 48–59 months (6.8%). Of the 366 children, 184 (50.3%) were female, and 182 (49.7%) were male. No significant association between age and undernutrition (wasting, stunting, and underweight) was detected ($p > 0.05$). Sex was significantly associated with stunting ($p = 0.028$). However, no significant association was detected between sex and wasting or being underweight. The highest percentage (83.9%) of mothers were between the ages of 21 and 35 years, the lowest percentage (7.9%) of the mothers were <20 years; 8.2% of mothers were >35 years, and the average age of mothers was 27 years.

The age of the mother was significantly associated with child stunting ($p = 0.042$). No significant association was detected between the age of the mother and wasting or underweight.

Table 1. Socio-demographic characteristics (n = 366)

Variables	Frequency	Percentage (%)
Age of child in month		
0 - 5	44	12
11-23	71	19.4
23-35	109	29.8
24 - 35	71	19.4
36 - 47	46	12.6
48 -59	25	6.8
Sex of child		
Female	184	50.3
Male	182	49.7
Age of mother		
< 20	29	7.9
21- 35	307	83.9
> 35	30	8.2
Educational status of mother		
Illiterate	30	8.2
Literate (Informal Education)	112	30.6
Primary School	114	31.1
Secondary	110	30.1
Family size		
≤ 5 members	265	72.4
≥ 6 members	101	27.6
Occupation of mother		
Agriculture	342	93.4
Public Servant	10	2.7
Business	11	3
Daily wage	3	0.8
Annual income in NPR		
RS. < 1.90 USD	115	31.4
RS. ≥1.90 USD	251	68.6

Nearly one-third of mothers completed informal education (30.6%); 31.1% completed primary schooling, 30.1% completed secondary schooling, and 8.2% were still illiterate. Education was not significantly associated with any form of undernutrition. A majority of the mothers were involved in agriculture (93.4%), followed by business (3%), public servants (2.7%), and daily wage workers (0.8%). The occupation was significantly associated with the prevalence of underweight children. A majority (72.7%) of the respondents lived together with five family members using the same cooking pot for at least six months; 27.6% lived with six family members. No relationship between family size and undernutrition was detected. Regarding income, 358 (97.8%) of the families were below the poverty line with an income of <1.90 USD/person/day. No significant association between income and undernutrition was detected.

Association of mother-related factors and undernutrition

The mother's age at the youngest childbirth was significantly associated with stunting ($p = 0.026$). No significant relationship between the age of the mother at the youngest childbirth and wasting or underweight was detected ($p > 0.05$). Postnatal check-ups during the postpartum period were significantly associated with underweight children ($p = 0.019$). However, there was no significant association between postnatal check-ups and wasting or stunting ($p > 0.05$). The use of modern contraceptives was significantly associated with underweight children ($p = 0.004$), whereas wasting and stunting were not significantly associated with the use of modern contraceptives. There was no significant association between alcohol consumption and being underweight ($p = 0.18$).

Discussion

This study was conducted in the marginalized indigenous Thami population of the Dolakha district of Nepal. The prevalence of undernutrition included 8.5% wasting (weight for height/length < −2 SD), 43.7% stunting (height for age < −2 SD), and 27.6% underweight. Stunting and underweight were more prevalent, whereas wasting was lower in our study than at the national level. According to the NDHS of 2016, the national prevalence rates for wasting, stunting, and underweight were 10%, 36%, and 27%, respectively (11). In our study, the prevalence of undernutrition was higher than in developing countries, which were 25% and 8.9% for stunting and wasting, respectively.

In our study, the prevalence of underweight children (27.6%) was less than in a similar study from 2017 in eastern Nepal of 37% (12). Among the malnourished children, 14.2% experienced severe stunting, and 6% were severely underweight; these prevalences were higher than the NDHS of 2016. No children were severely wasted in the present study. Furthermore, age-wise nutritional status, such as wasting, stunting, and underweight, was significantly higher during the second year of life, which may be due to a combination of interactive effects.

All three forms of undernutrition (wasting, stunting, and underweight) were higher in children between 12 and 23 months, similar to the 2016 NDHS. The prevalence of undernutrition was higher in males than females; 3.6% of females and 4% of males experienced wasting, 19.1% of females and 24.6% of males experienced stunting, 13.1% of females and 14.5% of males were underweight, similar to a previous study conducted in the Lamjung, Tanahu, and Gorkha districts in 2017 (13). The mother's age was significantly associated with stunting, similar to a study in Ghana (14).

Table 2. Pearson Chi-Square test for the association between socio-demographic characteristic and undernutrition

Veriables	Category	wasting			Stunting			Underweight		
		No	Yes	P value	No	Yes	P value	No	Yes	P value
Age of child in months	0 - 5	43	1	.073	24	20	.064	34	10	.786
		97.7%	2.3%		54.5%	45.5%		77.3%	22.7%	
	6 - 11	62	9		43	28		51	20	
		87.3%	12.7%		60.6%	39.4%		71.8%	28.2%	
	12 - 23	95	14		66	43		77	32	
		87.2%	12.8%		60.6%	39.4%		70.6%	29.4%	
	24 - 35	69	2		44	27		55	16	
		97.2%	2.8%		62.0%	38.0%		77.5%	22.5%	
	36 - 47	42	4		21	25		31	15	
		91.3%	8.7%		45.7%	54.3%		67.4%	32.6%	
	48 - 59	24	1		8	17		17	8	
		96.0%	4.0%		32.0%	68.0%		68.0%	32.0%	
Sex of Child	Female	171	13	.332	114	70	.028	136	48	.516
		92.9%	7.1%		62.0%	38.0%		73.9%	26.1%	
	Male	164	18		92	90		129	53	
		90.1%	9.9%		50.5%	49.5%		70.9%	29.1%	
Age of Mother	< 20	28	1	.395	14	15	.042	20	9	.241
		96.6%	3.4%		48.3%	51.7%		69.0%	31.0%	
	21- 35	281	26		181	126		227	80	
		91.5%	8.5%		59.0%	41.0%		73.9%	26.1%	
	> 35	26	4		11	19		18	12	
		86.7%	13.3%		36.7%	63.3%		60.0%	40.0%	
Family size using same cooking pot	≤ 5 members	240	25	.283	146	119	.457	70.2%	29.8%	.125
		90.6%	9.4%		55.1%	44.9%		79	22	
	≥ 6 members	95	6		60	41		78.2%	21.8%	
		94.1%	5.9%		59.4%	40.6%				
Educational status of mother	Illiterate	27	3	.786	12	18	.168	18	12	.350
		90.0%	10.0%		40.0%	60.0%		60.0%	40.0%	
	Literate	105	7		61	51		79	33	
		93.8%	6.3%		54.5%	45.5%		70.5%	29.5%	
	Primary School	103	11		71	43		86	28	
		90.4%	9.6%		62.3%	37.7%		75.4%	24.6%	
	Secondary	100	10		62	48		82	28	
		90.9%	9.1%		56.4%	43.6%		74.5%	25.5%	
Occupation of mother	Agriculture	314	28	.482	192	150	.163	248	94	.034
		91.8%	8.2%		56.1%	43.9%		72.5%	27.5%	
	Public Servant	9	1		6	4		8	2	
		90.0%	10.0%		60.0%	40.0%		80.0%	20.0%	
	Business	10	1		8	3		9	2	
		90.9%	9.1%		72.7%	27.3%		81.8%	18.2%	
	Daily wage	2	1		0	3		0	3	
		66.7%	33.3%		0.0%	100.0%		0.0%	100.0%	
Income per psrson per day	<1.90USD/ person/Day	202	156	.384	202	156	.717	258	100	.334
		56.4%	43.6%		56.4%	43.6%		72.1%	27.9%	
	≥ 1.90USD/ person/Day	4	4		4	4		7	1	
		50.0%	50.0%		50.0%	50.0%		87.5%	12.5%	

Table 3. Association between child related factors and undernutrition

Veriables	Category	wasting			Stunting			Underweight		
		No	Yes	P value	No	Yes	P value	No	Yes	P value
Weight of child at birth	<2.5 kg	14	1	.830	7	8	.263	12	3	.589
		93.3%	6.7%		46.7%	53.3%		80.0%	20.0%	
	≥2.5 kg	231	23		150	104		186	68	
		90.9%	9.1%		59.1%	40.9%		73.2%	26.8%	
Initiattion of breast feeding to child in hours	within one hour	272	26	.944	168	130	.941	216	82	.944
		91.3%	8.7%		56.4%	43.6%		72.5%	27.5%	
	after one hours	63	5		38	30		49	19	
		92.6%	7.4%		55.9%	44.1%		72.1%	27.9%	
Colostrum feeding to child immediately after birth	Yes	326	29	.240	200	155	.906	258	97	.509
		91.8%	8.2%		56.3%	43.7%		72.7%	27.3%	
	No	9	2		6	5		7	4	
		81.8%	18.2%		54.5%	45.5%		63.6%	36.4%	
Other food item fed immediately after child birth before breast feeding	Yes	14	2	.554	13	3	.040	13	3	.418
		87.5%	12.5%		81.3%	18.8%		81.3%	18.8%	
	No	321	29		193	157		252	98	
		91.7%	8.3%		55.1%	44.9%		72.0%	28.0%	
MR vaccination- I st	Yes	191	12	.146	120	83	.229	156	47	.032
		94.1%	5.9%		59.1%	40.9%		76.8%	23.2%	
	No	8	1		3	6		4	5	
		88.9%	11.1%		33.3%	66.7%		44.4%	55.6%	
Routine grouth monitoring	Yes	119	6	.002	79	46	.145	99	26	.098
		95.2%	4.8%		63.2%	36.8%		79.2%	20.8%	
	No	155	11		86	80		116	50	
		93.4%	6.6%		51.8%	48.2%		69.9%	30.1%	
Child getting sick within past two weeks	Yes	74	9	.377	41	42	.150	53	30	.048
		89.2%	10.8%		49.4%	50.6%		63.9%	36.1%	
	No	261	22		165	118		212	71	
		92.2%	7.8%		58.3%	41.7%		74.9%	25.1%	

The average family size of the studied community was 4.5, which is similar to national statistics. No significant association between education and wasting, stunting, or being underweight was detected, although 8.2%

of mothers were illiterate. Several studies demonstrated that higher maternal education lowered the prevalence of undernutrition (15, 16). However, education is not a single determinant of child undernutrition. The family size using the same cooking pot was significantly associated with undernutrition in this study, similar to another study conducted in Nepal (13). Almost 93% of mothers were involved in agriculture. Mothers' occupations were significantly associated with being underweight in this study, similar to a previous study carried out in 2018 in Ethiopia.

Family income is another important factor contributing to undernutrition. However, there was no significant relationship between income and undernutrition in this study, even though almost 97% of the families fell under the poverty line according to a recent cut-off point declared by the world bank (1.90 USD/person/day). In this study, the mother's age at first childbirth and postnatal check-ups were not significantly associated with undernutrition. However, age of mothers at last delivery (most recent), use of contraceptives, and extra food feeding before breastfeeding immediately after childbirth were significantly associated with stunting. Similarly, postnatal check-ups, vitamin A capsule intake in the postpartum period, use of contraceptives, and consumption of alcohol were significantly associated with being underweight.

CONCLUSION

Undernutrition is still a public health issue with a high prevalence among under-five children. The number of children in a family using the same cooking pot, the mother's age at the last delivery, contraceptive use, and introduction of other food items to children immediately after birth were significantly associated with stunting. Similarly, mothers' occupations, postnatal check-ups, intake of vitamin A capsules during the postpartum period, use of contraceptives, and consumption of alcohol during pregnancy were significantly associated with being underweight. These findings suggest that intervention of health risk behaviors is needed to reduce childhood undernutrition.

ACKNOWLEDGMENTS

The authors would like to acknowledge the College of Public Health Sciences, Chulalongkorn University, Thailand International Cooperation Agency (TICA), and the participants in this study. The authors declare that they have no conflict of interest.

REFERENCES

[1] UNICEF, WHO, Groups WB. Levels and trends in child nutrition. Key findings of the 2018 survey. URL: https://www.who.int/nutgrowthdb/2018-jme-brochure.pdf.

[2] WHO. Malnutrition 2018. URL: https://www.who.int/news-room/fact-sheets/detail/malnutrition.

[3] WHO. Malnutrition, key facts 2018. URL: https://www.who.int/news-room/fact-sheets/detail/malnutrition.

[4] WHO. World health statistics 2018. Geneva: WHO, 2018.

[5] Martins VJ, Toledo Florencio TM, Grillo LP, do Carmo PFM, Martins PA, Clemente AP, et al. Long-lasting effects of undernutrition. Int J Environ Res Public Health 2011;8(6):1817-46.

[6] Hume-Nixon M, Kuper H. The association between malnutrition and childhood disability in low- and middle-income countries: systematic review and meta-analysis of observational studies. Trop Med Int Health 2018;23(11):1158-75.

[7] Iliakis D, Kressig RW. [The relationship between malnutrition and immune]. Ther Umsch 2014;71(1):55-61.

[8] Sulaiman AA, Bushara SO, Elmadhoun WM, Noor SK, Abdelkarim M, Aldeen IN, et al. Prevalence and determinants of undernutrition among children under 5-year-old in rural areas: A cross-sectional survey in North Sudan. J Family Med Prim Care 2018;7(1):104-10.

[9] Statistics CBo. National population and housing census of Nepal, 2011. Kathmandu: Statistics CBo, 2012.

[10] Central Bureau of Statitics. National population and Housing Census 2011, Nepal. Kathmandu: Statistics CBo, 2012.

[11] MOHP. National Demographic Health survey 2016. Kathmandu: MOHP, 2017.

[12] Adhikari D, Khatri RB, Paudel YR, Poudyal AK. Factors associated with underweight among under-five Children in Eastern Nepal: Community-based cross-sectional study. Front Public Health 2017;5:350.

[13] Dhungana GP. Nutritional status and the associated factors in under five years children of Lamjung, Gorkha and Tanahun districts of Nepal. Nepal J Stat 2017;1:15-8.

[14] Wemakor A, Garti H, Azongo T, Garti H, Atosona A. Young maternal age is a risk factor for child undernutrition in Tamale Metropolis, Ghana. BMC Res Notes 2018;11(1):877.

[15] Abuya BA, Ciera J, Kimani-Murage E. Effect of mother's education on child's nutritional status in the slums of Nairobi. BMC Pediatrics 2012;12(1):80.

[16] Iftikhar A, Bari A, Bano I, Masood Q. Impact of maternal education, employment and family size on nutritional status of children. Pak J Med Sci 2017;33(6):1401-5.

Submitted: November 01, 2019. *Revised:* November 20, 2019. *Accepted:* November 27, 2019.

In: Pediatrics and Adolescent Health ISBN: 978-1-68507-490-6
Editors: J. Merrick and M. Morad

Chapter 6

WHAT ARE HONG KONG CHINESE PARENTS' PERCEPTIONS OF MATERIALISM AND EGOCENTRISM IN THEIR CHILDREN?

Daniel TL Shek[1,*], PhD, Lu Yu[1], PhD, Tak Yan Lee[2], PhD, Rachel CF Sun[3], PhD and Moon YM Law[4]

[1]Department of Applied Social Sciences, The Hong Kong Polytechnic University, Hong Kong, PR China
[2]Department of Social and Behavioral Sciences, City University of Hong Kong, Hong Kong, PR China
[3]Faculty of Education, The University of Hong Kong, Hong Kong, PR China
[4]Deparment of Social Work, The Chinese Univeristy of Hong Kong, Hong Kong PR China

[*] Corresponding Author's E-mail: daniel.shek@polyu.edu.hk.

Abstract

Although there are studies on adolescent materialism and egocentrism, most of them are Western studies based on the perspective of adolescents. As parents are significant others of adolescents, we investigated the perceptions of parents of materialism and egocentrism in their adolescent children as well as Hong Kong adolescents. Response frequency profiles generated from descriptive statistical analyses revealed that some parents perceived their children and adolescents in Hong Kong showing materialistic and egocentric concerns. However, consistent with the self-enhancement perspective, parents perceived their children to be less materialistic and egocentric than did Hong Kong adolescents in general. Several correlates of parents' perceptions of materialism and/or egocentrism in their children and adolescents in Hong Kong, including age, gender, and parental education, were identified in the current study.

Introduction

In different religious belief systems such as Christianity and Catholicism, the focus is on spiritual values such as faith, hope, and love instead of secular values such as hedonism and materialism. A similar focus on spiritual values is also found in other religious belief systems such as Buddhism and Taoism. However, with the rise of capitalism and consumerism in the past centuries, people begin to attach great importance to material possession and money. The tendency to focus on material possession is commonly referred to as materialism. According to Belk (1), materialism refers to the importance of "worldly possessions" (p. 291) to an individual which is characterized by three maladaptive features, including the tendency to possess (i.e., possessiveness), lack of generosity (i.e., non-generosity) and envy of the possessions of others. Similarly, Richins (2) defined materialism as "the importance ascribed to the ownership and acquisition of material goods in achieving life goals or desired states" (p. 210). From Maslow's hierarchy of needs (3), while material possession can help an individual to fulfill physical needs as well as security needs, materialism is not directly related to belongingness need, esteem needs, and self-actualization needs.

According to Shek and Siu (4), materialism is an unhealthy traditional cultural value in the Chinese culture, as reflected in some cultural beliefs such as "xiao pin bu xiao chang" (it is more shameful about being poor than being a prostitute), "you qian neng shi gui tui mo" (money makes the devil push the millstone), "ren qiong zhi duan" (poverty stifles ambition), and "pin ju nao shi wu ren wen, fu zai shen shan you yuan qin" (no one cares about a poor man even if he lives downtown, while distant relatives visit a rich man even if he lives in a remote mountain). In contemporary Hong Kong, as it is an international financial center, money and material possession are commonly regarded as legitimate life goals chased by people. Obviously, over-emphasis on materialism can be regarded as a risk factor which would impair the development of Chinese adolescents.

Empirically, studies showed that adolescents held materialistic beliefs. Based on the responses of 1,658 high school students, Shek, Ma, and Lin (5) showed that high proportions of the respondents agreed that "I believe that money is everything", "my life goal is to earn as much money as possible", "the amount of money one makes is a fundamental indicator of one's success", and "I believe that money makes the mare go". Similarly, in the studies of Shek and Lin (6) and Shek and other colleagues (7) that examined materialism in 2,474 Chinese high school students based on the perspective of adolescents, they found that high proportions of respondents regarded that "money is everything", "possessing money or consumer goods would make one happy", and "one's life goal is to earn as much money as possible". However, adolescents perceived their materialism to be lower than that of Hong Kong adolescents in general. Similarly, based on the perceptions of 568 teachers, many teachers agreed that their students and adolescents in Hong Kong regarded earning money was more important than other things (8, 9). Interestingly, teachers saw their students to be less materialistic than did adolescents in the general population.

Developmentally, over-emphasis on materialism in adolescence has two negative consequences. First, this would lead to unbalanced and distorted adolescent development with a darkening of spiritual values.

For example, when adolescents place important emphasis on material possession, they would not regard voluntary service to be important. Adolescents would also place instrumental value on interpersonal relationships. Actually, in many adolescent developmental models and personality theories, the focus on youth development is commonly placed on virtues and non-material developmental goals (10, 11, 12, 13, 14). Second, materialism leads to heightened stress in adolescents who are struggling for upward social mobility and survival. There are findings showing that while materialism was positively related to egocentrism, materialistic beliefs are negatively related to morality, spirituality, and empathy (5).

According to Shek and Siu (4), another unhealthy value faced by adolescents in Hong Kong is egocentrism. According to Elkind (15), egocentrism is a natural developmental phenomenon. With cognitive maturity (i.e., reaching formal operation stage in Piagetian theory, [16]), self-consciousness in adolescents increases but differentiation between oneself and others is lacking where adolescent egocentrism is characterized by focus on self, belief that other people also focus on themselves, perception that one is unique, and belief that one's views and experience are superior than others (17, 18). Egocentrism in Hong Kong young people are shaped by traditional Chinese cultural beliefs, such as the popular saying of "ren bu wei ji, tian zhu di mie" (Heaven destroys those who do not look out for themselves). It is also influenced by contemporary Hong Kong culture, exemplified by the cultural saying of "ni you ni yao qiu, wo you wo gan shou" (you have your own requests and I have my own experiences). Empirically, there are research findings showing that egocentrism impairs adolescent developmental outcomes. In Shek, Yu, and Siu's (18) study, they showed that adolescent egocentrism was positively related to materialism but negatively related to morality and empathy.

In the study based on the responses of 1,658 high school students, findings showed that many students showed signs of egocentrism: around nine-tenth of the students felt that their experiences are different from others, more than half of the respondents believed that their views are better than those of others, and roughly one-third believed that their benefits are more important than others (18). In another study based on the responses of 2,474 high school students, students perceived that themselves and adolescents in Hong Kong, in general, showed signs of egocentrism: roughly one-fifth of junior high school students perceived themselves as always finding excuses for their behavior; roughly one-quarter of senior high school students perceived that they could always find excuses for their behavior. The students also saw themselves as less egocentric than did adolescents in Hong Kong in general (6). Shek and colleagues (9) also conducted another study examining teachers' perceptions of materialism and egocentrism in adolescents in Hong Kong. Based on the responses of 568 teachers, findings showed that the respondents generally saw their students showing signs of egocentrism: around 84% of their students believed that their experiences are more important than others; around 46% of their students believed that others' criticisms of their behavior are groundless; 77% of the students believed that their experience is more important than others. Similarly, very high proportions of the teachers perceived that adolescents in Hong Kong showed egocentrism: around 90% of young people believed that their experiences are more important than the experience of others; 87.4% of adolescents in Hong Kong believed that their benefits are more important than benefits of other people; 87% of the adolescents in Hong Kong can always find excuses for their behavior. However, teachers perceived that materialism and egocentrism in their students were lower than those of Hong Kong adolescents.

As far as data collection is concerned, most of the existing studies are based on adolescents' perspectives. This is not desirable because social desirability effect is intrinsic to self-report amongst adolescents. For example, in the studies of Shek and colleagues (7) and Shek and Ma (8), results showed that adolescents saw themselves and Hong Kong adolescents to be less materialistic and egocentric compared to teachers' perceptions of materialism and egocentrism in their students and adolescents in Hong Kong. Obviously, understanding how other people look at materialism and egocentrism in adolescents would be of paramount importance to triangulate the findings based on adolescents alone.

Besides teachers, it would be desirable to understand the perceptions of parents on materialism and egocentrism in adolescents in Hong Kong. There are two reasons why we should understand parents' perceptions of materialism and egocentrism in their children and adolescents in general. First, as significant others of their adolescent children, parents spend much time with them. As such, parents may have an in-depth understanding of materialism and egocentrism in their children. Such an understanding may also help parents to have good knowledge of adolescents in Hong Kong. Second, compared with adolescents, parents may have more skills in understanding and analyzing the behavior of their children and adolescents. Third, there are numerous studies showing that parents exert a strong influence on adolescent development (19, 20). Hence, it would be theoretically and practically important to understand parents' perceptions of materialism and egocentrism in their adolescent children and adolescents in general.

In view of the importance of understanding materialism, egocentrism, and psychosocial development in Hong Kong adolescents, a series of studies were conducted with the support of the Wofoo Foundation (6, 8, 21, 22, 23). To understand the related phenomena in a holistic manner, we collected data from adolescents, teachers, and parents to triangulate the findings. Besides the studies based on adolescents (7) and teachers (9), we also conducted a study looking at materialism and egocentrism based on the perceptions of parents (21).

In this paper, we present findings on parents' perceptions of adolescent materialism and egocentrism with reference to several objectives. First, we investigated Chinese parents' perceptions of materialistic and egocentric characteristics of high school students and adolescents in Hong Kong. By looking at the profiles of responses, we can understand the materialistic and egocentric issues in young people in Hong Kong from the perspective of parents. Second, we addressed the research question of whether parental perceptions of materialism and egocentrism differed between their children and adolescents in general in

Hong Kong. Based on the literature on social psychology, it was hypothesized that compared to adolescents in general, adolescent children would be seen by their parents as less materialistic and egocentric. Third, as previous studies showed that there are socio-demographic correlates of students' and teachers' perceptions of materialism and egocentrism in high school students and adolescents (7, 9), we also investigated whether there are socio-demographic correlates of parents' perceptions of materialism and egocentrism in their children and adolescents in general.

OUR STUDY

To examine the views of parents on adolescent materialism and egocentrism, we recruited 431 parents (mean age = 44.57) from nine secondary schools in Hong Kong. As it is not easy to engage parents in surveys, the number of parents participating in this study can be regarded as respectable. The parents were invited to complete a self-report questionnaire which covers different aspects of psychosocial development of their adolescent children and adolescents in Hong Kong, including materialism, egocentrism, moral character, and other social behavior. For each parent randomly selected from a family, a self-report questionnaire was sent to the parent who completed the questionnaire in a self-administered manner. The completed questionnaire was then put in a sealed envelope in an anonymous manner and returned to the school. Approval from the University Institutional Review Board was obtained before the commencement of the study. School consent as well as parental consent were obtained before data collection.

Instruments

Parents' Perception of Adolescent Materialism

Based on the abridged 5-item Chinese Adolescent Materialism Scale (5), we developed a scale to assess parents' perception of materialistic beliefs in Chinese adolescents. These items included: a) "my children believe that making money is more important than any other things"; b) "My children believe that money is everything"; c) "My children believe that the rich can get respect from others"; d) "My children would abandon some principles for the sake of money"; and e) "My children believe that the amount of money one makes is a fundamental indicator of one's success". For each item, there are six response options, including "strongly disagree", "disagree", "slightly disagree", "slightly agree", "agree", and "strongly agree", with higher scores indicating higher levels of materialism in their adolescent children.

The five items used in Shek, Ma, and Lin (5) were used to assess parents' perceptions of materialistic beliefs amongst Hong Kong adolescents in general. The items included: a) "Hong Kong adolescents think that making money is more important than any other things"; b) "Hong Kong adolescents believe that money is everything"; c) "Hong Kong adolescents think that the rich can get respect from others"; d) "Hong Kong adolescents would abandon some principles for the sake of money"; and e) "Hong Kong adolescents believe that the amount of money one makes is a fundamental indicator of one's success". These items are measured on a 6-point scale, with higher scores reflecting higher levels of perceived materialism in Hong Kong adolescents.

Parents' Perception of Adolescent Egocentrism

We used the simplified 5-item Chinese Adolescent Egocentrism Scale (18) to assess parental perceptions of egocentrism in their children and Hong Kong adolescents. These items included: a) "My children regard their experiences are more important than those of others"; b) "My children think that their interests are more important than those of others"; c) "My children always find justifications for their behavior"; d) "most of the time, my children think that other people's criticisms about them do not make sense"; e) "even if they make other people are unhappy, my children are true to their experience". A 6-point scale, with "strongly disagree", "disagree", "slightly disagree", "slightly agree",

"agree", and "strongly agree" as the response options were used. Higher scale scores suggest higher levels of egocentrism.

For parents' perceptions of adolescent egocentrism, we used the abridged 5-item Chinese Adolescent Egocentrism Scale (6, 18). These items included: a) "Hong Kong adolescents regard their experiences are more important than those of others"; b) "Hong Kong adolescents think that their interests are more important than those of others"; c) "Hong Kong adolescents always find justifications for their behavior"; d) "most of the time, Hong Kong adolescents think that other people's criticisms about them do not make sense"; e) "even if they make other people are unhappy, Hong Kong adolescents are true to their experience". There are six response options in each item, with higher scores indicating higher levels of perceived egocentrism in adolescents in Hong Kong.

Data analyses

With respect to the objectives of the study, several lines of analyses were performed. First, descriptive statistical analyses were conducted to examine the response profiles of the parents to the different scales. By focusing on the percentage findings, we can understand the concerns of materialism and egocentrism in parents' adolescent children and Chinese adolescents. Second, we examined parents' perceptions of the egocentrism and egocentrism in their children and see whether they differed from the related responses based on Hong Kong adolescents. Based on the previous findings (6, 9), we expected that parents would see their children to be less materialistic and egocentric than do adolescents in general. Third, we conducted analyses to examine the related socio-demographic correlates. Several general expectations were put forward. First, as older people are more traditional and conservative, they might see adolescents to be more materialistic and egocentric. Second, as females are more accommodating and tolerant, they would see adolescents to be less materialistic and egocentric. Third, as parents with more education know young people more, they would see adolescents to be more materialistic and egocentric.

FINDINGS

Table 1. Parent perception of materialistic beliefs in their own children

Items	1	2	1+2	3	4	5	4+5	Mean	n
	n	n	n	n	n	n	n		
	(%)	(%)	(%)	(%)	(%)	(%)	(%)		
1. My children believe making money is more important than any other things.	87 (20.2%)	151 (35.1%)	238 (55.3%)	107 (24.9%)	77 (17.9%)	8 (1.9%)	85 (19.8%)	2.46	430
2. My children believe "Money is everything".	138 (32.3%)	162 (37.9%)	300 (70.3%)	69 (16.2%)	53 (12.4%)	5 (1.2%)	58 (13.6%)	2.12	427
3. My children believe "No money, no dignity".	128 (30.1%)	127 (29.9%)	255 (60.0%)	87 (20.5%)	73 (17.2%)	10 (2.4%)	83 (19.6%)	2.32	425
4. My children believe they would abandon some principles for the sake of money.	244 (57.4%)	115 (27.1%)	359 (84.5%)	42 (9.9%)	22 (5.2%)	2 (0.5%)	24 (5.6%)	1.64	425
5. My children believe "The amount of money one makes is a fundamental indicator of one's "success".	118 (27.7%)	138 (32.4%)	256 (60.1%)	93 (21.8%)	66 (15.5%)	11 (2.6%)	77 (18.1%)	2.33	426

Based on the percentage findings, we could examine the response profiles of parents' views of materialism and egocentrism in their adolescent children and adolescents in Hong Kong. The related findings are outlined in Table 1 to Table 4. First, some parents perceived their adolescent children to be materialistic: roughly one-fifth of the parents believed that "my children believe making money is more important than any other things" and "my children believe that there is no dignity if there is no money". Second, many parents perceived that Hong Kong adolescents showed signs of materialism: nearly 45% of the parents perceived that "adolescents in Hong Kong believed that there is no dignity if there is no money"; roughly 42% of the parents perceived that "adolescents in Hong Kong believed the amount of money one makes is a fundamental indicator of one's success". Third, many parents perceived their children to be egocentric: 47% of the parents saw that "my children believe their feelings are more important than the feelings of other people; roughly 54% of the parents believed that "my children believe that no matter what happens, they can always justify their behavior". Fourth, a majority of the parents perceived that Hong Kong adolescents, in general, showed signs of egocentrism: "adolescents in Hong Kong believed their feelings are more important than the feelings of other people" (66.7%); "adolescents in Hong Kong believed that no matter what happens, they can always justify their behaviors" (71.8%); "adolescents in Hong Kong are loyal to their own feelings even if this may upset other people" (61.7%).

To compare perceived materialism in parent's children and adolescents in Hong Kong, several independent t-tests were conducted. Findings showed that the parents saw their children to be less materialistic than did adolescents in Hong Kong on the individual items and composite scores (Table 5). Similarly, we compared perceived egocentrism in the respondents' children and youths in Hong Kong. Again, findings showed that parents' perception of egocentrism in adolescents in Hong Kong was higher than did parents' own adolescent children (Table 6).

Pearson correlation analyses showed that parental age was positively related to materialism in their own children and egocentrism in Hong Kong adolescents. Mothers also saw their children and Hong Kong adolescents to be less materialistic. Parental education was also positively related to materialism in Hong Kong adolescents and egocentrism in their children and adolescents in Hong Kong (see Table 7).

Table 2. Parent perception of materialistic beliefs in Hong Kong adolescents

Items	1	2	1+2	3	4	5	4+5	Mean	n
	n	n	n	N	n	n	n		
	(%)	(%)	(%)	(%)	(%)	(%)	(%)		
1. Adolescents in HK believe making money is more important than any other things.	38 (8.9%)	113 (26.5%)	151 (35.4%)	114 (26.7%)	142 (33.3%)	20 (4.7%)	162 (38.0%)	2.98	427
2. Adolescents in HK believe "Money is everything".	55 (12.9%)	111 (26.0%)	166 (38.9%)	109 (25.5%)	124 (29.0%)	28 (6.6%)	152 (35.6%)	2.90	427
3. Adolescents in HK believe "No money, no dignity".	42 (9.9%)	94 (22.2%)	136 (32.1%)	98 (23.1%)	148 (34.9%)	42 (9.9%)	190 (44.8%)	3.13	424
4. Adolescents in HK believe they would abandon some principles for the sake of money.	88 (20.8%)	103 (24.3%)	191 (45.0%)	123 (29.0%)	95 (22.4%)	15 (3.5%)	110 (25.9%)	2.64	424
5. Adolescents in HK believe "The amount of money one makes is a fundamental indicator of one's "success".	37 (8.6%)	87 (20.3%)	124 (29.0%)	123 (28.7%)	143 (33.4%)	38 (8.9%)	181 (42.3%)	3.14	428

Regression analyses were also conducted to identify the predictors of perceived materialism in their children. Compared with fathers, mothers perceived their children to be less materialistic (Table 8). Regarding perceived materialism in Hong Kong adolescents, parental gender and parental education were significant predictors. Compared to fathers, mothers saw adolescents in Hong Kong to be less materialistic; parents with lower educational attainment also saw Hong Kong adolescents to be less materialistic (Table 9). For perceived egocentrism in the children, there was no significant predictor (Table 10). In contrast, age and parental education were positively related to perceived egocentrism in adolescents in Hong Kong (Table 11).

Table 3. Parent perception of egocentrism in their own children

Items	1 n (%)	2 n (%)	1+2 n (%)	3 n (%)	4 n (%)	5 n (%)	4+5 n (%)	Mean	n
1. My children believe their feelings are more important than the feelings of other people.	33 (7.7%)	97 (22.6%)	130 (30.2%)	98 (22.8%)	155 (36.0%)	47 (10.9%)	202 (47.0%)	3.20	430
2. My children believe their own benefits are more important than the benefits of other people.	62 (14.5%)	137 (32.1%)	199 (46.6%)	116 (27.2%)	102 (23.9%)	10 (2.3%)	112 (26.2%)	2.67	427
3. My children believe that no matter what happens, they can always justify their behaviors.	38 (8.9%)	65 (15.3%)	103 (24.2%)	95 (22.3%)	171 (40.1%)	57 (13.4%)	228 (53.5%)	3.34	426
4. My children believe the criticisms on them are usually groundless.	36 (8.5%)	130 (30.6%)	166 (39.1%)	133 (31.3%)	104 (24.5%)	22 (5.2%)	126 (29.6%)	2.87	425
5. My children are loyal to their own feelings even if this may upset other people.	48 (11.2%)	108 (25.1%)	156 (36.3%)	117 (27.2%)	124 (28.8%)	33 (7.7%)	157 (36.5%)	2.97	430

Table 4. Parent perception of egocentrism in Hong Kong adolescents

Items	1	2	1+2	3	4	5	4+5	Mean	n
	n (%)	n (%)	n (%)	n (%)	n (%)	n (%)	n (%)		
1. Adolescents in HK believe their feelings are more important than the feelings of other people.	15 (3.5%)	55 (12.9%)	70 (16.4%)	72 (16.9%)	202 (47.3%)	83 (19.4%)	285 (66.7%)	3.66	427
2. Adolescents in HK believe their own benefits are more important than the benefits of other people.	22 (5.2%)	49 (11.5%)	71 (16.6%)	101 (23.7%)	189 (44.3%)	66 (15.5%)	255 (59.7%)	3.53	427
3. Adolescents in HK believe that no matter what happens, they can always justify their behaviors.	12 (2.8%)	45 (10.6%)	57 (13.5%)	65 (15.3%)	205 (48.2%)	98 (23.1%)	303 (71.8%)	3.78	425
4. Adolescents in HK believe the criticisms on them are usually groundless.	14 (3.3%)	67 (15.8%)	81 (19.1%)	107 (25.2%)	181 (42.7%)	55 (13.0%)	236 (55.7%)	3.46	424
5. Adolescents in HK are loyal to their own feelings even if this may upset other people.	15 (3.5%)	57 (13.4%)	72 (16.9%)	91 (21.4%)	179 (42.0%)	84 (19.7%)	263 (61.7%)	3.61	426

Table 5. Differences in materialistic beliefs between own children and HK adolescents perceived by parents

	Children	**HK Adolescents**	*t*	*p*
1. My children/HK adolescents believe that...	*M*	*M*		
2. Making money is more important than any other things	2.46	2.98	-8.64	.000
3. Money is everything.	2.12	2.90	-12.41	.000
4. No money, no dignity.	2.32	3.13	-13.51	.000
5. They would abandon some principles for the sake of money.	1.64	2.64	-16.86	.000
6. The amount of money one makes is a fundamental indicator of one's "success".	2.33	3.14	-13.94	.000
Composite Score	2.18	2.96	-17.29	.000

Note. $p < .05$; The result is significant; The performance of own children is better than HK adolescents perceived by parents.

Table 6. Differences in egocentrism between own children and HK adolescents perceived by parent

	Children	**HK Adolescents**	*t*	*p*
1. My children/HK adolescents believe that...	*M*	*M*		
2. Their feelings are more important than the feelings of other people.	3.20	3.66	-8.31	.000
3. Their own benefits are more important than the benefits of other people.	2.67	3.53	-15.95	.000
4. Not matter what happens, they can always justify their behaviors.	3.34	3.78	-8.26	.000
5. The criticisms on them are usually groundless.	2.87	3.46	-11.25	.000
6. They are loyal to their own feelings even if this may upset other people.	2.97	3.61	-11.21	.000
Composite Score	3.01	3.61	-15.04	.000

Note. $p < .05$; The result is significant; The performance of own children is better than HK adolescents perceived by parents.

Table 7. Correlation among variables

Variables	1	2	3	4
1. Age	-			
2. Gender[a]	-0.184***	-		
3. CSSA[b]	0.028	-0.010	-	
4. Parental Education[c]	0.074	-0.104*	0.125**	-
5. Materialism in own children	0.100*	-0.130**	-0.070	0.076
6. Materialism in HK adolescents	0.073	-0.096*	0.069	0.243***
7. Egocentrism in own children	-0.001	-0.016	0.020	0.092*
8. Egocentrism in HK adolescents	0.107*	-0.039	0.008	0.260***

Note. *p <.05, **p <.01, ***p <.001.

[a]Male = 1, Female = 2; [b]Receiving CSSA = 1, Not receiving CSSA = 2.

[c]Primary and below = 1, Secondary = 2, Above secondary = 3.

Table 8. Predicting effects of demographic factors on parent perceived materialism in their own children

Predictors	Materialism in own children			
	β	t	F	R^2
Age	0.082	1.672	2.794	0.007
Gender[a]	-0.120	-2.486*	6.180*	0.014
CSSA[b]	-0.078	-1.609	2.589	0.006
Parental Education[c]	0.053	1.103	1.217	0.003

Note. *p <.05, **p <.01, ***p <.001.

[a]Male = 1, Female = 2; [b]Receiving CSSA = 1, Not receiving CSSA = 2.

[c]Primary and below = 1, Secondary = 2, Above secondary = 3.

Table 9. Predicting effects of demographic factors on parent perceived materialism in HK adolescents

Predictors	Materialism in HK adolescents			
	β	t	F	R^2
Age	0.062	1.276	1.629	0.004
Gender[a]	-0.100	-2.073*	4.298*	0.010
CSSA[b]	0.060	1.231	1.515	0.004
Parental Education[c]	0.239	5.068***	25.683***	0.057

Note. *p <.05, **p <.01, ***p <.001.

[a]Male = 1, Female = 2; [b]Receiving CSSA = 1, Not receiving CSSA = 2.

[c]Primary and below = 1, Secondary = 2, Above secondary = 3.

Table 10. Predicting effects of demographic factors on parent perceived egocentrism in their own children

Predictors	Egocentrism in own children			
	β	*t*	*F*	R^2
Age	0.000	-0.004	0.000	0.000
Gender[a]	-0.022	-0.448	0.201	0.000
CSSA[b]	0.020	0.419	0.176	0.000
Parental Education[c]	0.076	1.577	2.486	0.006

Note. *p <.05, **p <.01, ***p <.001.
[a]Male = 1, Female = 2; [b]Receiving CSSA = 1, Not receiving CSSA = 2.
[c]Primary and below = 1, Secondary = 2, Above secondary = 3.

Table 11. Predicting effects of demographic factors on parent perceived egocentrism in Hong Kong adolescents

Predictors	Egocentrism in HK adolescents			
	β	*t*	*F*	R^2
Age	0.103	2.105*	4.430*	0.011
Gender[a]	-0.500	-1.030	1.061	0.003
CSSA[b]	0.014	0.278	0.078	0.000
Parental Education[c]	0.260	5.543***	30.722***	0.068

Note. *p <.05, **p <.01, ***p <.001;
[a]Male = 1, Female = 2; [b]Receiving CSSA = 1, Not receiving CSSA = 2;
[c]Primary and below = 1, Secondary = 2, Above secondary = 3

CONCLUSION AND DISCUSSION

The present study examined parents' perceptions of materialism and egocentrism in their adolescent children and adolescents in Hong Kong. There are three unique features of this study. First, as most of the studies have been based on self-report from adolescents, the employment of parents as respondents in this study is a pioneer in the field. Second, we examined parents' perceptions of their children and Hong Kong adolescents in general which can give a more dynamic picture about materialism and egocentrism in young people in Hong Kong. Third, we attempted to identify the socio-demographic correlates of perceived materialism and egocentrism amongst adolescent children and Hong Kong adolescents in general in Hong Kong which have not been explored in previous studies.

Regarding the response profiles of the respondents, two phenomena were observed. First, while some parents perceived their children as materialistic, many more parents perceived that Hong Kong adolescents were materialistic. Second, many parents perceived their children and adolescents in Hong Kong to be egocentric. These observations are consistent with those reported previously based on the perspective of adolescents (6, 9) and teachers (8, 9).

Consistent with our expectation, parents perceived that their children were less materialistic than did Hong Kong adolescents in general. Similarly, parents perceived their children to be less egocentric as compared to Hong Kong adolescents in general. These observations are in line with the previous findings in the social psychological literature on self-enhancement that people tend to see themselves (or people related to themselves) to be more favorable than people in the outgroup (24).

Several observations can be highlighted from the findings based on the regression analyses on the socio-demographic correlates of perceived materialism and egocentrism beliefs in Chinese adolescents. First, compared with fathers, mothers perceived a lower level of materialism in their children as well as adolescents in Hong Kong. This may be explained by the fact that mothers are more accommodating and tolerant than do fathers. Parental education was also found to be a significant predictor of perceived materialism in Hong Kong adolescents. This may be explained in terms of the exposure of the parents where those with higher education would have a better understanding of adolescents in Hong Kong. For perceived adolescent egocentrism, there was no significant socio-demographic correlate of perceived egocentrism in their own children. However, age and parental education were positively associated with perceived egocentrism in adolescents in Hong Kong. As people with higher age might be more traditional and conservative, they would see adolescents in Hong Kong as more egocentric.

Again, those with higher education attainment may have a better understanding of adolescents in Hong Kong, hence having a more negative view of egocentrism in adolescents.

As no study has been conducted to understand materialism and egocentrism in adolescents based on the perspective of parents, the present findings are pioneer in nature. Nevertheless, it is noteworthy that there are several limitations of the present study. First, the sample was based on the convenience sampling method only. Hence, we have to replicate the findings and use random samples in future. Second, there are five items in the assessment of materialism and five items in the assessment of egocentrism. As such, employment of longer scales assessing different aspects of these two aspects would be helpful. Third, the findings on the socio-demographic correlates are tentative only. Therefore, further refinement and strengthening of the conceptual bases of the hypotheses would be helpful. Finally, as parents play an important role in the socialization of materialism in adolescents (25-29), it would be helpful to examine parental influences further. It would also be theoretically and practically important to understand how parents contribute to the development of materialism and egocentrism in adolescents in future studies.

ACKNOWLEDGMENTS

The series of studies on character and moral development in high school students in Hong Kong are financially supported by Wofoo Foundation. This chapter is a re-published version of an earlier paper: Shek DTL, Yu L, Lee TY, Sun RCF, Law MYM. What are Hong Kong Chinese parents' perceptions of materialism and egocentrism in their children? *International Journal of Child and Adolescent Health* 2020;13(3):229-39.

REFERENCES

[1] Belk RW. Three scales to measure constructs related to materialism: Reliability, validity, and relationships to measures of happiness. Adv Consum Res 1984;11:291-7.

[2] Richins ML. The material values scale: Measurement properties and development of a short form. J Consum Res 2004;31:209-19303-16.

[3] Maslow AH. *Motivation and personality*. New York: Harper Row, 1954.

[4] Shek DTL, Siu AMH. "UNHAPPY" Environment for adolescent development in Hong Kong. J Adolesc Health 2019;64(6):S1-S4. doi:10.1016/j.jadohealth.2019.01.007

[5] Shek DTL, Ma CMS, Lin L. The Chinese Adolescent Materialism Scale: Psychometric properties and normative profiles. Int J Disabil Hum Dev 2014;13(2):285-95.

[6] Shek DTL, Lin L. A study on the development of Chinese students (Character, psychosocial competence and behavior): Report No. 1 – Views of students. Hong Kong: Department of Applied Social Sciences, The Hong Kong Polytechnic University, 2017.

[7] Shek DTL, Lin L, Siu AMH, Lee B. Materialism in Chinese adolescents in Hong Kong: Profiles and socio-demographic correlates. Int J Child and Adolesc Dev, in press.

[8] Shek DTL, Ma CMS. A study on the development of Chinese students (Character, psychosocial competence and behavior): Report No. 2 – Views of teachers. Hong Kong: Department of Applied Social Sciences, The Hong Kong Polytechnic University, 2017.

[9] Shek DTL, Ma CMS, Siu AMH, Lee B. Materialism and egocentrism in Chinese adolescents in Chinese adolescents in Hong Kong: Perceptions of teachers. Int J Child Adolesc Health, in press.

[10] Shek DTL, Dou D, Zhu X, Chai W. Positive youth development: Current perspectives. Adolesc Health Med Ther 2019;10:131-41. doi:10.2147/AHMT.S179946

[11] Frankl V. Man's search for meaning. London: Vintage Publishing, 2004.

[12] Park N. Building strengths of character: Keys to positive youth development. Reclaiming Child Youth 2009;18(2):42-7.

[13] Park N, Peterson C. Moral competence and character strengths among adolescents: The development and validation of the values in action inventory of strengths for youth. J Adolesc, 2006;29:891-909.

[14] Catalano RF, Berglund ML, Ryan JAM, Lonczak HS, Hawkins JD. Positive youth development in the United States: Research findings on evaluations of positive youth development programs. Ann Am Acad Pol Soc Sci 2004;591(1):98-124. doi:10.1177/0002716203260102

[15] Elkind D. Egocentrism in adolescence. Child Dev 1967;38:1025-34.

[16] Piaget J. Judgment and reasoning in the child. London: Routledge & Kegan Paul, 1972.

[17] Elkind D, Bowen R. Imaginary audience behavior in children and adolescents. Dev Psychol 1979;15:38–44.

[18] Shek DTL, Yu L, Siu AMH. The Chinese Adolescent Egocentrism Scale: Psychometric properties and normative profiles. Int J Disabil Hum Dev 2014;13(2):297-307. doi:10.1515/ijdhd-2014-0315.

[19] Shek DTL, Zhu X, Ma CMS. The influence of parental control and parent-child relational qualities on adolescent internet addiction: A 3-year longitudinal study in Hong Kong. Front Psychol 2018;9:642. doi:10.3389/fpsyg.2018.00642.

[20] Shek DTL, Zhu X, Dou D. Influence of family processes on internet addiction among late adolescents in Hong Kong. Front Psychiatry 2019;10:113. doi:10.3389/fpsyt.2019.00113.

[21] Shek DTL, Yu L. A study on the development of Chinese students (Character, psychosocial competence and behavior): Report No. 3 – Views of parents. Hong Kong: Department of Applied Social Sciences, The Hong Kong Polytechnic University, 2018.

[22] Shek, DTL, Leung J. A study on the development of Chinese students (Character, psychosocial competence and behavior): Report No. 4 – Moral education at the crossroad. Hong Kong: Department of Applied Social Sciences, The Hong Kong Polytechnic University, 2018.

[23] Shek DTL, Wu FKY, Leung H. A study on the development of Chinese students (Character, psychosocial competence and behavior): Report No. 5 – A qualitative study of the views of principals and teachers on moral education. Hong Kong: Department of Applied Social Sciences, The Hong Kong Polytechnic University, 2018.

[24] Dunning D. Self-insight: Roadblocks and detours on path to knowing thyself. New York: Psychology Press, 2005.

[25] Huta V. Linking peoples' pursuit of eudaimonia and hedonia with characteristics of their parents: Parenting styles, verbally endorsed values, and role modeling. J Happiness Stud 2012;13(1):47-61. doi:10.1007/s10902-011-9249-7

[26] Huta, V. Eudaimonic and hedonic orientations: Theoretical considerations and research findings. In J. Vittersø eds. Handbook of eudaimonic well-being. International handbook of quality of life. Cham, Switzerland: Springer, 2016:215-31.

[27] Huta V, Ryan RM. Pursuing pleasure or virtue: The differential and overlapping well-being benefits of hedonic and eudaimonic motives. J Happiness Stud 2010;11(6):735-62.

[28] Huta V, Waterman AS. Eudaimonia and its distinction from hedonia: Developing a classification and terminology for understanding conceptual and operational definitions. J Happiness Stud 2014;15:1425-56. doi:10.1007/s10902-013-9485-0

[29] Huta V, Pelletier LG, Baxter D, Thompson A. How eudaimonic and hedonic motives relate to the well-being of close others. J Posit Psychol 2012;7(5):399-404.

In: Pediatrics and Adolescent Health ISBN: 978-1-68507-490-6
Editors: J. Merrick and M. Morad

Chapter 7

HOUSING RISK FACTORS ASSOCIATED WITH DIARRHEA AND PNEUMONIA AMONG CHILDREN RESIDING IN AN URBAN SLUM IN ENUGU METROPOLIS, NIGERIA

Joy Nkeiruka Ozughalu*
Institute of Public Health, College of Medicine,
University of Nigeria, Enugu Campus, Nigeria

ABSTRACT

Childhood diarrhea and pneumonia are among the leading causes of morbidity and mortality in children under five years of age, accounting for over two million deaths annually worldwide. The main objective of this study was to identify the housing risk factors associated with diarrhea and pneumonia in children less than five years living in the Ngenevu slum area of Enugu Metropolis, Nigeria. A community-based cross-sectional study was adopted and an interviewer administered questionnaire was employed to elicit response from mothers/caregivers residing in selected households with at least one under-five child. This

*Corresponding Author's E-mail: joyozughalu@yahoo.co.uk.

study employed a multistage sampling technique. This study found the prevalence of diarrhea and pneumonia to be 38.8% and 24.7% respectively. In multivariate analysis, educational level of mothers/caregivers, number of under five years children living in households, method of disposal of child's feces and source of drinking water were significantly associated with diarrhea. Knowledge about pneumonia, ventilation status and exclusive breastfeeding practices were found statistically significant with pneumonia ($P \leq 0.05$). Improvement in housing conditions, sanitation/hygienic practices, exclusive breastfeeding in the first six months of life would markedly reduce morbidity and mortality in children under five years from diarrhea and pneumonia diseases.

INTRODUCTION

Housing is universally acknowledged as one of the most basic human needs after food. In modern concept, housing is not limited only to the physical structure serving as shelter, but also the immediate environment including community services and facilities (1). The housing situation in Nigeria is unsatisfactory and grossly inadequate both in numerical terms and in qualitative aspects (2). This shortfall has led to substandard living conditions affecting the quality of life of the majority of the populace, especially children.

Trends in global disease burden have shown that attention in health outcomes has shifted from severe morbidity to psychosocial wellbeing in the developed countries (3), but for developing countries like Nigeria, high morbidity and mortality rates from infectious diseases rather than chronic/lifestyle diseases is still the main focus. According to the WHO factsheets, an estimated 6.3 million children under the age of 15 years died in 2017 and of these, 5.4 million were under five years of age with over 50 per cent of these under five years deaths occurring in Africa (4). This translates into 15,000 under five years deaths per day, globally. About 80 per cent of these deaths occur in sub-Saharan Africa and South Asia, with Nigeria being among the six countries that account for half of these under five years deaths (4). These worrisome figures are due to conditions that are preventable and treatable with simple and affordable interventions.

Among the leading causes of death in children under five years are pneumonia, diarrhea and malaria, which are preventable and treatable through implementable interventions (5).Pneumonia and diarrhea account for 29% of all child deaths, leading to the loss of more than two million young lives each year. Most child deaths from pneumonia and diarrhea occur in the world's poorest regions – with nearly 90% in sub-Saharan Africa and South Asia (5). The burden that pneumonia and diarrhea places on families and health systems in low-resource countries further widens existing inequalities.

Risk factors for these disease outcomes include overcrowded conditions, indoor air pollution, unsanitary conditions, unsafe drinking water and food and poor hygiene practices which are highly connected to poor housing conditions. Nigeria is one of the most densely populated countries in the world with daunting challenges in the provision of affordable and adequate housing. Enugu State, a state in the eastern part of Nigeria, with an urban growth rate of 2.5% and an urban population of about 927,642 residents is faced with high housing needs to cater for this influx of people (6, 7).

Despite various government led interventions and global efforts that have been implemented to address high morbidity and mortality rates among underfives, the menace is still unabated. Based on this fact, the significance of this study lies in its ability to identify relevant housing risk factors of diarrhea and pneumonia in under five years children in the study location which will further direct and guide interventions from both governmental and non-governmental organizations. Also, findings from this study would strongly harp on the need for quick redirection and implementation of already formulated policies that will improve the health outcomes of children under five years (in particular) living in urban slums in Enugu metropolis and other low-income settlements in the Nigerian state. This study is novel as no such study, to the best of the researcher's knowledge has been carried out in any urban slum in Enugu State, not even in the southeastern part of Nigeria. The objectives of this study include: to ascertain the level of mothers'/caregiver's knowledge, identify the influence of housing conditions, sanitation/hygienic factors, breastfeeding practices/immunization statuses on the occurrence of diarrhea and respiratory tract diseases (pneumonia) among underfives residing in Ngenevu slum area in Enugu Metropolis.

OUR STUDY

A community based cross-sectional study was carried out in selected households with children less than five years of age residing in Ngenevu urban slum. Enugu North Local Government Area (LGA) is one of the seventeen local government areas in Enugu State and also one of the three local government areas that make up Enugu urban, capital of Enugu State. It has a total area of about 106km^2, a total population of 244,852 and a female population of 123,227 extracted from the National Population Census of 2006. Enugu North LGA is made up of seven localities; of these seven localities, major slums can be found in three localities namely, Iva-valley, Ogbete and Ogui new layout. Ogbete houses the second most populated urban slum- Ngenevu slum area- in Enugu metropolis. The housing patterns are haphazard with no defined streets or housing numbers (8).

This study was carried out over a period of two weeks in June, 2019. The sample size was determined using this statistical formula, $n = Z^2 p(1-p)/d^2$, where n = required sample size, Z = confidence level of 95% (1.96), p = assuming a population proportion/prevalence rate (0.5), d = degree of precision or accuracy expressed as a proportion 0.05, which is 5%. The total sample size of 422 was gotten after 10% non-response rate consideration.

Households who were eligible for inclusion in the study had the presence of a mother or female caregiver with at least one child under the age of five and have resided in the area for at least six months and consented to participate while mothers/caregivers who have hearing and/or speech disabilities and those who withheld their consent to participate were excluded. This study employed a multistage sampling technique. Enugu North Local Government Area was selected using simple random sampling. out of the LGAs that make up Enugu Metropolis, Out of the seven localities (Iva-valley, GRA, New Haven, Asata, Ogbete, Ogui New Layout and Independence layout) making up Enugu North, Ogbete locality was selected using simple random sampling. Selection of households from Ogbete locality (Ogbete central ward) which houses Ngenevu urban slums were done randomly from the already zoned areas of the slum and systematically selecting households to ensure proper randomization considering the scattered and haphazard nature of houses (8).

A well-structured modified questionnaire was developed using the National Demographic and Health Survey template as appropriate to address study objectives. Interviewer administered questionnaire was employed to elicit responses from mothers/caregivers residing in selected households with at least one under-five child with the aid of two trained research assistants that underwent a 2-day training session on the objectives of the study, techniques of face-to-face interview, how to approach respondents and how to keep confidentiality among other things. Data collection was supervised by the chief researcher for consistency and completeness of data. Approval was gotten from the Health Research and Ethics Committee, University of Nigeria Teaching Hospital, Ituku-Ozalla. Informed consent was also sought and obtained from mothers/caregivers after detailed explanation on the purpose of study. Any involvement of the mother was after their complete consent.

Definition of variables

Childhood diarrhea, which is an outcome/dependent variable was defined as having three or more watery stools in 24 hours in the previous four weeks preceding the study.

Pneumonia, also an outcome variable was measured based on the WHO criteria for pneumonia which is having a cough and/or fast breathing and difficulty in breathing (9).

Others are the independent variables which include: family size, mother's/caregiver's age, child's age and gender, educational status, occupation, number of children under five years in the household, mother's/caregiver's knowledge on the childhood diseases, housing and environmental factors, breastfeeding and immunization statuses. These variables are defined accordingly.

The level of mother's/caregiver's knowledge on diarrhea and pneumonia occurrence in their underfive children was ascertained from their responses to questions bordering on; having heard about diarrhea or pneumonia, their signs and symptoms, their causes and danger signs. An affirmative answer to each of these questions earn the respondent a high level of knowledge and if otherwise, a low level of knowledge on the occurrence of childhood diarrhea and pneumonia. Overcrowding status was ascertained if the number of persons living in a room was less than or equal to two (Not overcrowded) or if number of persons living in a room was greater than two (Overcrowded).

Ventilation status was gotten from a combination of variables. Firstly, if the number of windows per room is greater than two, then it is considered as good ventilation, if it is less than or equal to two, then it is designated as poor ventilation. Secondly, if the major type of cooking fuel was electricity or liquefied gas, then it is good ventilation, if kerosene or wood or charcoal was used as major cooking fuel and cooking is done in a separate building or outdoors, it is good ventilation. Cooking done inside the household with kerosene or wood or charcoal is termed poor ventilation.

Satisfactory toilet facility was gotten if toilet was not shared with other households and type of toilet was flush toilet but if toilet is shared with other household and type of toilet facility is not flush toilet then it is unsatisfactory. Satisfactory place of child defecation was gotten if child defecated in the flush toilet, in a potty or in his/her diaper and non-satisfactory if child defecated on the floor. Disposal of child feces was proper if disposed in the toilet, other methods of disposal were deemed improper. Hand washing with water and soap (proper hand washing method) and hand washing with water alone (Improper method). Respondents who washed their hands always; after using the toilet, disposal of child feces, before and after food preparation and feeding of child had adequate frequency in hand washing, other respondents who did not always wash their hands before or after these activities had inadequate frequency in hand washing. Dumpsite was regarded as the only proper place for garbage disposal, other places or methods were improper. Disposal of wastewater into sewage system was proper while disposal of wastewater into streets or nearby shallow gutters were improper.

Buying of food from street vendors (always, usually or sometimes) by respondents for their children under five years was termed unacceptable child feeding practice while respondents who never bought food from street vendors had acceptable child feeding practice. If source of drinking water was piped into homes, from public taps, boreholes and sachet water then it is termed adequate but if source of drinking water was from dug well or tanker trucks then it was inadequate. If time to get drinking water was less than 30 minutes (round trip) or water is within dwelling, then time to get water was optimal and if more than 30 minutes, it was suboptimal.

Breastfeeding practice was defined in terms of exclusive breastfeeding and not exclusively breastfed. Immunization statuses were defined based on mother's/caregivers response on completion or non-completion of child's immunization schedule.

Data analysis

Data were analyzed using Statistical Package for the Social Sciences (SPSS) Version 25. Descriptive statistics was computed whereby proportion/percentages and frequency was calculated. Cross tabulation and Pearson's chi-square test were computed to establish the association between the dependent and independent variables. Variables that were significant at $p \leq 0.05$ after bivariate analysis were further plugged into multivariate logistic analysis to obtain the adjusted odds ratio. Copies of questionnaire with incomplete responses were excluded before analyses were carried out.

FINDINGS

The majority of the respondents 211 (54.9%) were within the age group 26-34 years, while only four (1.0%) within age group 44-52 years. Of the children, females (53.1%) participated more in this study. Educational level with the highest frequency was secondary level with 256 (66.7%) respondents. Three hundred and forty two respondents were married while 130 respondents were self-employed (see Table 1).

Table 1. Frequency distribution of socio-demographic variables

Category	Frequency (n=384)	Percentage (%)
Age of Respondents (Years)		
17-25	129	33.6
26-34	211	54.9
35-43	40	10.4
44-52	4	1.0
Age of Child (Months)		
1-15	259	67.4
16-30	97	25.3
31-45	17	4.4
46-60	11	2.9
Gender of Child		
Male	180	46.9
Female	204	53.1
Educational Level of Respondents		
No Education	7	1.8
Primary level	63	16.4
Secondary level	256	66.7
Tertiary level	58	15.1

Category	Frequency (n=384)	Percentage (%)
Marital Status		
Married	342	89.1
Single	24	6.3
Widowed	8	2.1
Divorced	5	1.3
Separated	5	1.3
Occupation		
Self Employed	130	33.9
Petty Trader	117	30.5
Housewife	67	17.4
Civil servant	53	13.8
Student	17	4.4
No. of underfives in households.		
1	152	39.6
2	164	42.7
3	55	14.3
4	11	2.9
5	2	5.0

Source: Computed by author.

Frequency distribution for the dependent variables

Table 2 shows that out of the 384 respondents who had under five years old children, 149 (38.8%) had diarrhea in the preceding four weeks leading to this study, while 235 (61.2%) did not have diarrhea. Also, out of 384 respondents with underfive children, 94 (24.7%) experienced symptoms of pneumonia in the preceding four weeks prior to the study while 290 (75.3%) did not.

Table 2. Frequency distribution for the dependent variables

Diarrhea Outcome	Frequency	Percent (%)
Present	149	38.8
Absent	235	61.2
Total	384	100.0
Pneumonia Outcome	**Frequency**	**Percent (%)**
Present	94	24.7
Absent	290	75.3
Total	384	100.0

Source: Computed by author.

Socio-demographic variables versus Diarrhea outcome

Children within age group1-15months had the highest diarrhea outcome (39.8%). Males (40.0%) had higher outcome of diarrhea. Highest outcome of diarrhea were seen in mothers/caregivers with no education (71.4%), divorced (60.0%), petty trader (43.6%), and households with four under five years children (63.6%).Educational status and number of under five years children in household were statistically significant with diarrhea outcomes at 5% level of significance (P=0.000 respectively) while age of child, gender of child, occupation of mother/caregiver and marital status were not statistically significant (see Table 3).

Table 3. Socio-demographic variables versus diarrhea outcome

Variables	Diarrhea occurrence		P-values	Odds ratio	95%	
	Present (%)	Absent (%)			Confidence	Interval
					Lower	Upper
Age group of						
child 1-15 months	103 (39.8)	156 (60.2)				
16-30 months	37(38.1)	60(61.9)	0.407	0.882	0.657	1.196
31-45 months	5(29.4)	12(70.6)				
46-50 months	4(36.4)	7(63.6)				
Gender						
Male	72 (40.0)	108 (60.0)				
Female	77 (37.7)	127 (62.3)	0.651	0.909	0.603	1.372
Educational level						
No education	5 (71.4)	2 (28.6)				
Primary level	42 (66.7)	21 (33.3)	0.000	0.864	0.817	0.915
Secondary level	90 (35.2)	166 (64.8)				
Tertiary level	12 (20.7)	46 (79.3)				
Marital status						
Single	6 (25.0)	18 (75.0)				
Married	136 (39.8)	206 (60.2)				
Divorced	3 (60.0)	2 (40.0)	0.640	1.097	0.745	1.615
Widowed	2 (25.0)	6 (75.0)				
Separated	2 (40.0)	3 (60.0)				
Occupation						
Civil servant	14 (26.4)	39 (73.6)				
Self employed	55 (42.3)	75 (57.7)				
Housewife	27 (40.3)	40 (59.7)	0.586	1.051	0.879	1.256
Petty Trader	51 (43.6)	66 (56.4)				
Student	2 (11.8)	15 (88.2)				

Variables	Diarrhea occurrence		P-values	Odds ratio	95% Confidence	Interval
	Present (%)	Absent (%)			Lower	Upper
No of underfive in households						
One	44 (28.9)	108 (71.1)				
Two	65 (39.6)	99 (60.4)				
Three	32 (58.2)	23 (41.8)	0.000	1.666	1.254	2.161
Four	7 (63.6)	4 (36.4)				
Five	1 (50.0)	1 (50.0)				

Source: Computed by author.

Socio-Demographic variables and Pneumonia occurrence

As shown in Table 4, pneumonia outcome was slightly higher in females (24.5%) than in males (24.4%). Children within the age group 31-45 months had the highest pneumonia outcome at approximately 53%. Respondents with no educational background had the highest percentage (57.1%) of underfives who had experienced pneumonia. and this association was statistically significant. (P=0.013).

Table 4. Socio-demographic variables and pneumonia occurrence

Variables	Pneumonia occurrence		P value	Odds ratio	95% Confidence Interval	
	Present	Absent			Lower bound	Upper bound
Age group of child						
1-15 months	58 (22.4)	201 (77.6)				
16-30 months	25 (25.8)	72 (74.2)	0.163	1.245	0.915	1.695
31-45 months	9 (52.9)	8 (47.1)				
46-50 months	3 (18.2)	9 (81.8)				
Gender						
Male	44 (24.4)	136 (75.6)				
Female	50 (24.5)	154 (75.5)	0.912	0.974	0.612	1.550
Educational level						
No education	4 (57.1)	3 (42.9)				
Primary level	23 (36.5)	40 (63.5)	0.013	0.931	0.880	0.985
Secondary level	55 (21.5)	201 (78.5)				
Tertiary level	12 (20.7)	46 (79.3)				

Table 4. (Continued)

Variables	Pneumonia occurrence		P value	Odds ratio	95% Confidence Interval	
	Present	Absent			Lower bound	Upper bound
Marital status						
Single	6 (25.0)	18 (75.0)				
Married	86 (25.1)	256 (74.9)				
Divorced	0 (0.0)	5 (100.0)	0.374	0.800	0.490	1.307
Widowed	1 (12.5)	7 (87.5)				
Separated	1 (20.0)	4 (80.0)				
Occupation						
Civil servant	9 (17.0)	44 (83.0)				
Self employed	33 (25.4)	97 (74.6)				
Housewife	13 (19.4)	54 (80.6)	0.303	1.112	0.909	1.360
Petty Trader	37 (31.6)	80 (68.4)				
Student	2 (11.8)	15 (88.2)				
No of underfive in household						
One	33 (21.7)	119 (78.3)				
Two	47 (28.7)	117 (71.3)				
Three	10 (18.2)	45 (81.8)	0.857	1.066	0.805	1.411
Four	4 (36.4)	7 (63.6)				
Five	0 (0.0)	2 (100.0)				

Source: Computed by author.

Highest outcome of pneumonia was seen in under five year olds whose mothers were married (25.1%), petty trader (31.6%) and had four under five years children living in the households (36.4%). Analysis between the dependent variable (pneumonia occurrence) and socio-demographic variables such as age of child, gender of child, marital status, occupation and number of children under five years of age in households showed no statistical significance.

Knowledge on diarrhea and pneumonia in underfives versus dependent variables

Among the respondents 215 (56.0%) had good knowledge of diarrhea, while 169 (44.0%) had low knowledge of diarrhea. Of the 384 respondents only 32 (8.3%) had good knowledge of pneumonia while 352(91.7%) had low knowledge of pneumonia (see Table 5). Analysis between the dependent variable-occurrence of diarrhea in the past four weeks-and knowledge of diarrhea showed that 42.3% of respondents who had good knowledge of diarrhea and 34.3% who had low knowledge had had their children suffer from diarrhea. Further analysis using chi-square test showed no significant association between these two variables at 5% level of significance.

Analysis on the variables pneumonia symptoms and knowledge of pneumonia as seen in Table 5 showed that 37.5% of under five years children with pneumonia outcomes were seen among respondents with good knowledge of pneumonia while 23.3% of children with pneumonia outcome were seen among those with low knowledge of pneumonia. This variable showed statistical significance. (P=0.030).

Table 5. Knowledge on diarrhea and pneumonia in underfive versus dependent variables

Diarrhea outcome				
Good Knowledge of Diarrhea	Frequency (n=384) & Percent (%)	Present (%)	Absent (%)	P-value and χ^2 value
Yes	215 (56.0)	91 (42.3)	124 (57.7)	P=0.110
No	169 (44.0)	58 (34.3)	111(65.7)	χ^2= 2.554
Pneumonia outcome				
Good Knowledge of Pneumonia	Frequency (n=384) & Percent (%)	Present (%)	Absent (%)	P-value and χ^2 value
Yes	32 (8.3)	13 (37.5)	19 (62.5)	P=0.030
No	352 (91.7)	81 (23.3)	271 (76.7)	χ^2=4.731

Source: Computed by author.

Housing variables (crowding and ventilation statuses) and pneumonia outcome

Of the 384 households sampled as shown in Table 6, 332 (86.5%) were overcrowded, 329 (85.7%) had poor ventilation status and 55 (14.3%) had satisfactory ventilation status. Analysis between pneumonia symptoms and crowding status showed that out of 332 overcrowded households, 87 (26.5%) of them had their children coming down with pneumonia while out of 52 non-overcrowded households, 7 (13.5%) of them had their children experienced pneumonia symptoms. Chi-square analysis indicates a significant association at 5% level of significance. P= 0.043.Results from analysis also indicated that 5.5% of under five years old who had experienced pneumonia in the past four weeks lived in households whose overall ventilation status was satisfactory while 28.4% of underfives lived in households with poor ventilation status. Chi-square test showed significant association between these two variables at 5%. P=0.000 (see Table 6).

Table 6. Housing variables (crowding and ventilation statuses) and pneumonia outcome

Pneumonia outcome				
Overcrowding Status	Frequency (n=384) & Percent (%)	Present (%)	Absent (%)	P value & χ^2 value
Overcrowded	332 (86.5)	87 (26.5)	245 (73.5)	P=0.043
Not overcrowded	52 (13.5)	7 (13.5)	45(86.5)	χ^2= 4.109
Overall Ventilation Status	Frequency (n=384) & Percent (%)	Present (%)	Absent (%)	P value & χ^2 value
Satisfactory	55 (14.3)	3 (5.5)	52(94.5)	P=0.000
Non satisfactory	329 (85.7)	91 (28.4)	238 (71.6)	χ^2=12.823

Source: Computed by author.

Sanitation/hygienic factors versus diarrhea outcome

Descriptive statistics between occurrence of diarrhea and toilet facilities showed that out of 149 underfive years old with diarrhea outcome 133

(38.8%) resided in households with unsatisfactory toilet facilities and 16 (39.0%) had satisfactory toilet facilities. Pearson's chi-square test showed no significant relationship between these two variables at 5% (see Table 7).

For the variable place of child defecation, out of 149 underfives who had diarrhea, 25 (48.1%) lived in households with no satisfactory place of child defecation while 124 (37.3%) lived in households with satisfactory place of child defecation. There was no significant relationship between occurrence of diarrhea and place of child defecation. (P= 0.140).For the variable disposal of faeces, 104 (45.0%) out of 149 underfive children with diarrhea resided in households without satisfactory place of disposal of child's faeces compared to 45 (29.4%) of underfive year old children with diarrhea who had satisfactory place of disposal. There exists significant association between occurrence of diarrhea and place of disposal of faeces at 5% level of significance. P= 0.002 (see Table 7).

Table 7. Sanitation/hygienic factors versus diarrhea outcome

Variables	**Frequency (n=384) & Percent (%)**	**Diarrhea Outcome**		**P value & χ^2 value**
		Present (%)	Absent (%)	
Satisfactory Toilet Facilities				
Yes	191(49.7)	16 (39.0)	25 (61.0)	P= 0.975
No	193(50.3)	133 (38.8)	210 (61.2)	χ^2= 0.001
Satisfactory Place of Child Defecation				
Yes	337(87.8)	124 (37.3)	208 (62.7)	P= 0.140
No	47(12.2)	25 (48.1)	27 (51.9)	χ^2= 2.179
Satisfactory Disposal of Faeces				
Yes	161(41.9)	45 (29.4)	108 (70.6)	P= 0.002
No	223 (58.1)	104 (45.0)	127 (55.0)	χ^2= 8.445
Frequency of Hand washing				
Satisfactory	164(42.7)	59 (36.2)	104 (63.8)	P= 0.368
Non satisfactory	220(57.3)	90 (40.7)	131 (59.3)	χ^2=0.810
Proper Hand washing				
Yes	102(26.5)	29 (28.4)	73 (71.6)	P= 0.012
No	282(73.5)	120 (42.6)	162 (57.4)	χ^2= 4.219
Proper Disposal of Garbage				
Yes	154(40.1)	45 (31.9)	96 (68.1)	P= 0.035
No	230(59.9)	104 (42.8)	139 (57.2)	χ^2= 4.451

Table 7. (Continued)

Variables	Frequency (n=384) & Percent (%)	Diarrhea Outcome		P value & χ^2 value
		Present (%)	Absent (%)	
Proper Disposal of Wastewater				
Yes				
No	23(6.0)	9 (39.1)	14 (60.9)	P= 0.973
	361(94.0)	140 (38.8)	221 (61.2)	χ^2=0.001
Acceptable Feeding Practice				
Yes	121 (31.5)	46 (38.0)	75 (62.0)	P= 0.830
No	263 (68.5)	103 (39.2)	160 (60.8)	χ^2= 0.046
Adequate Source of Drinking Water				
Yes	268 (69.8)	92 (34.3)	176 (65.7)	P= 0.006
No	116 (30.2)	57 (49.1)	59 (50.9)	χ^2= 4.255
Optimal Time to get Drinking Water				
Yes	298 (77.6)	117 (39.3)	181(60.7)	P= 0.731
No	86 (22.4)	32 (37.2)	54 (62.8)	χ^2= 0.118

Source: Computed by author.

Results for frequency of hand washing showed that 90 (40.7%) of mothers of underfive year olds with diarrhea outcome had a non-satisfactory frequency of hand washing compared to 59(36.2%) mothers with underfives with diarrhea outcome who had satisfactory frequency of hand washing. Pearson's chi-square test showed no significant association between occurrence of diarrhea and frequency in hand washing at 5%. P=0.368. For the variable, hand washing practice and occurrence of diarrhea, analysis showed that 120 (42.6%) mothers who did not practice proper hand washing had their child suffer from diarrhea in the past four weeks compared to 29 (28.4%) mothers who practiced proper hand washing. A significant association also exists between hand washing practice and diarrhea occurrence in underfives within the past four weeks. P= 0.012.

Descriptive statistics between diarrhea occurrence and disposal of garbage showed that 104 (42.8%) of under five years old who came down with diarrhea in the preceding four weeks came from households with improper disposal of garbage compared to 45 (31.9%) with proper disposal of garbage. Frequency distribution on method of garbage disposal revealed that majority of the household burnt and open-dumped their garbage. Pearson's Chi-square analysis indicated a significant relation between disposal of garbage and diarrhea occurrence (P=0.035).Children who had diarrhea 140 (38.8%) were from households that lack proper disposal of wastewater, nine (39.1%) came from houses with proper method of disposing wastewater. The association between household method of disposal of wastewater and diarrhea occurrence showed no statistical significance (P= 0.973) (see Table 7).

Diarrhea occurrence and feeding practice was analyzed and results as displayed in Table 7 showed that 103 (39.2%) mothers whose children came down with diarrhea had non-acceptable feeding practice compared to 46 (38.0%) mothers whose children came down with diarrhea had acceptable feeding practice. There was no significant relationship between diarrhea outcome and feeding practice (i.e., buying of foods from street vendors) P=0.830. Approximately 49% of under five years old children with diarrhea resided in households with inadequate source of drinking water compared to 34.3% who were from households with adequate source of drinking water. Analysis using Pearson chi-squared test showed a significant association between source of drinking water and diarrhea outcome at 5% level of significance. P=0.006. Time to get drinking water was also not significantly related to diarrhea outcome (P=0.731; OR=0.917, CI 0.559-1.504), as 32 (37.2%) of households who had suboptimal time to get drinking water had underfives with diarrhea outcome compared to 117(39.3%) of households who had optimal time to get drinking water.

Breastfeeding/immunization practice and the dependent variables

Table 8 shows that 261 (68%) of respondents did not exclusively breastfeed their children in the first six months of life, while 123 (32.0%) respondents breastfed their children exclusively. Of the 384 respondents,

221 (57.6%) had immunized their underfive years old children against measles while 163 (42.4%) had not immunized their children against measles. Three hundred and seventy one (96.6%) had not received rotavirus vaccine, while only 13 (3.4%) had received rotavirus vaccine.

Table 8. Breastfeeding/immunization practice and the dependent variables

Breastfeeding/Immunization Practice and Diarrhea Outcome				
Variables	**Frequency (n=384) & Percent (%)**	**Diarrhea outcome**		**P value & χ^2 value**
		Present (%)	Absent (%)	
Exclusively Breastfed (First six month)				
Yes	123 (32.0)	39 (30.0)	84 (70.0)	P= 0.017
No	261(68.0)	110(42.8)	151 (57.2)	χ^2= 5.695
Measles Immunization				
Yes	221(57.6)	87 (38.9)	134 (61.1)	P= 0.792
No	163 (42.4)	62 (38.6)	101 (61.4)	χ^2= 0.070
Rotavirus Immunization				
Yes	13 (3.4)	2 (15.4)	11 (84.6)	P= 0.545
No	371(96.6)	147 (39.1)	224 (60.9)	χ^2= 0.366
Breastfeeding/Immunization Practice and Pneumonia Outcome				
Variables	**Frequency (n=384) & Percent (%)**	**Pneumonia Outcome**		**P value &χ^2 value**
		Present (%)	Absent (%)	
Exclusively Breastfed (First six month)				
Yes	123 (32.0)	21 (16.7)	102 (83.3)	P= 0.013
No	261(68.0)	73(28.4)	188 (71.6)	χ^2= 6.110
Measles Immunization				
Yes	221(57.6)	54 (24.4)	167 (75.6)	P= 0.872
No	163 (42.4)	40 (25.2)	123 (74.8)	χ^2= 0.026

Source: Computed by author.

One hundred and ten (42.8%) of underfive years old with diarrhea outcome were not exclusively breastfed compared to 39 (30.0%) who came down with diarrhea though exclusively breastfed. This association was statistically significant at 5%. P= 0.017. There was slight difference in proportion between those who were given measles vaccine and those not given measles vaccine, but came down with diarrhea, (38.9 and 38.6) respectively. This association was statistically insignificant at 5%. P=0.792. Rotavirus immunization showed no statistical significance with diarrhea occurrence. P= 0.545. Out of 13 underfive year olds who had received rotavirus vaccine, two (15.4%) came down with diarrhea compared to 147 (39.1%) who had not received rotavirus vaccine and came down with diarrhea (see Table 8).

Analysis between pneumonia occurrence and exclusive breastfeeding in underfive years children showed that pneumonia was absent in 83.3% of under five years who were breastfed in their first six month of life. A significant relationship at 5% level of significance exists. (P=0.013). Also, 75.6% of under five years old in whom pneumonia was absent had been immunized against measles. There was no significant association between pneumonia occurrence and measles vaccination in under five years old (P=0.872).

Multivariate logistic regression analysis of the variables

After carrying out multivariate analysis with the dependent variable – diarrhea outcomes, and other independent variables, risk factors that were significant includes; Educational level (P=0.000, AOR=0.879, 95%CI=0.828-0.933), Number of underfive children living in households (P=0.001, AOR=1.593, 95%CI=1.207-2.102),Method of disposal of child's feces (P=0.005, AOR=0.512, 95%CI=0.321-0.817), and source of drinking water (P=0.008, AOR=0.521, 95%CI=0.322-0.842).

The result as displayed in Table 9 shows that after the dependent variable – Pneumonia outcome was plugged in with other independent variables. Knowledge of Pneumonia (P=0.002, AOR=3.959, 95%CI=1.671-9.380), Ventilation status (P=0.004, AOR=0.171, 95%CI=0.051-0.576) and Exclusive breastfeeding at first six month (P=0.040, AOR=0.546, 95%CI=0.307-0.971) emerged significant at 5% level.

Table 9. Multivariate logistic regression analysis between the two outcome variables and other independent variables

Dependent variable – Diarrhea outcome				
Independent Variables	**5% Significant level**	**Adjusted (Odds ratio)**	**95% Confidence Interval**	
			Upper bound	Lower bound
Educational level	0.000	0.879	0.828	0.933
No of children U5 in household	0.001	1.593	1.207	2.102
Disposal of child faeces	0.005	0.512	0.321	0.817
Hand washing practice	0.129	0.654	0.378	1.132
Disposal of household garbage	0.392	0.807	0.493	1.319
Sources of drinking water	0.008	0.521	0.322	0.842
Exclusive breastfeeding at first six month of life	0.243	0.739	0.445	1.227
Dependent variable – Pneumonia outcome				
Independent Variables	**5% Significant level**	**Adjusted (Odds ratio)**	**95% Confidence Interval**	
			Upper bound	Lower bound
Educational level	0.114	0.951	0.894	1.012
Knowledge of pneumonia	0.002	3.959	1.671	9.380
Overcrowding	0.181	0.544	0.223	1.327
Overall ventilation status	0.004	0.171	0.051	0.576
Exclusive breastfeeding at first six month of life	0.040	0.546	0.307	0.971

Source: Computed by author.

DISCUSSION

This study provides the prevalence of childhood diarrhea and pneumonia and their associated risk factors in the previous four weeks preceding collection of data. This study found out that prevalence of diarrhea in under five years children was 38.8% and the prevalence of pneumonia was 24.7%. These results show that diarrhea and pneumonia are highly prevalent among underfives residing in Ngenevu slum area. The prevalence of childhood diarrhea and pneumonia is quite high compared to studies carried out by Sanya and Stanly (10), (7.6% and 12.2%) and

Chaturvedi et al. (11), (11.9% and 15.5%). This discrepancies may be due to the fact that this study was carried out in a slum area where all indices for quality standard of living is low with high level of exposure to risk factors, not also ruling out variations in case definitions and data collectors skill.

Analysis from socio demographic variables showed that children within 1-15months of age had the highest outcome of diarrhea. Though not statistically significant, this finding is similar to study carried out in Rwanda, where children within the age group 1-12months had the highest outcome of diarrhea (12). Among the socio- demographic variables, the key predictors for diarrhea among under five years old children were educational level of mothers/caregivers and number of children under the age of five years living in households. The under five years old children with mothers/caregivers with no education and those with primary education had the highest outcome of diarrhea 71.4% and 66.7% respectively. Odds ratio analysis revealed that as educational level increases the odds of diarrhea decreases (OR=0.879, 95%CI=0.828-0.933). This finding is similar to findings from Nsabimana, Mureithi and Habiu (12) and Yilgwan and Okolo (13).The education level of the mother is likely to positively affect household hygienic practices, enhance approach to child health care and decision making at critical times.

This study showed that diarrhea was significantly associated with the presence of two or more under five years children living in the same household. This study also found out that the odds of having diarrhea increased as the number of children increased in a particular household. This finding is in agreement with studies by Mengistie, Berhane and Worku (14) as well as Yilgwan and Okolo (13). The more children under five years living in the same household is a predictor for diarrheal diseases. Children at this stage get in contact with potential disease causing agents and the probability of cross contamination becomes high among children living in a confined space.

Analysis between socio-demographic variables and pneumonia showed that educational level was a key predictor for pneumonia occurrence. The odds of children under five years contracting pneumonia reduces with an increase in mothers' educational level. Education creates awareness and increases alertness towards health care choices and outcomes. This finding is supported by Gritly et al. (15) in their study carried out in a Sudanese hospital, which purported that a high proportion of pneumonia prevailed among children whose mother had lower education. Ujunwa and Ezeonu (16) also found significant association between poor parental education and pneumonia. On the contrary, Fekadu, Terefe and Aleme (17) in a community based study found no significant association between pneumonia and parental education.

On the level of mothers'/caregivers' knowledge on diarrhea, findings from this study showed that there was good knowledge of diarrhea (56.0%) among respondents, but this knowledge did not transform into proper practices that would have prevented against diarrhea occurrence in their children. Approximately 42% of children under five years with diarrhea were from mothers with very high knowledge of diarrhea compared to 34.3% of those that had mothers with poor knowledge. However, this association was statistically insignificant. Frequency distribution showed a low level of knowledge of mothers/caregivers on pneumonia occurrence. Only 8.3% of respondents had appropriate knowledge of pneumonia. The majority of the respondents alluded that pneumonia was caused by cold weather. Bivariate and multivariate analysis between these two variables showed statistical significance at 5% level of significance. This study found that the odds of a child under five years coming down with pneumonia increased in mothers with good knowledge of pneumonia. Good knowledge of mothers with regard to pneumonia outcome was not protective against pneumonia, possibly because of the overwhelming contaminated environment and a high probability that mothers who reported in the affirmative of their children having pneumonia were those who were able to recognize the signs and symptoms, causes and danger signs correctly. This implies that there may be children under five years of age that had pneumonia in the preceding four weeks, but were not reported in this study due to the inability of their mothers to recognize the signs and symptoms, causes and danger signs of pneumonia.

At the level of bivariate analysis, this study found that housing condition (crowding and ventilation status) was significantly associated with childhood pneumonia. More than 86% of the households were overcrowded and 85.7% had non-satisfactory ventilation. The number of persons per room in these households far exceeded the stipulated standards defined by this study thus leading to overcrowding. In support of this finding, 26.5% of pneumonia outcomes were in overcrowded households compared to 13.5% from non-overcrowded households. Fekadu, Terefe and Aleme (17) indicated that crowding status is an important determinant factor of pneumonia occurrence.

Exposure to indoor and outdoor pollutants has been linked to pneumonia occurrence. Findings from the study area revealed that most households used unclean fuel both for cooking and lighting activities. These cooking fuels, especially solid fuels like wood and charcoal emits poisonous irritants into the air thereby reducing household air quality. Fekadu, Terefe and Aleme (17) found an association between the use of charcoal as cooking fuel and pneumonia occurrence. Most households visited do their cooking outdoors, but the proximity to sleeping areas is not significant to prevent indoor air pollution. Number of windows per room in the majority of the slum households was inadequate and in some cases, sizes were inappropriate. More than twenty-eight percent of pneumonia outcomes were in household with non-satisfactory ventilation compared to 5.5% in households with satisfactory ventilation. On further analysis using multivariate regression model, ventilation status of households alone was statistically significant and the odds of pneumonia occurrence in children under five years was 83% less likely in households with satisfactory ventilation. (OR=0.171) In agreement to the findings of this study, Nirmola et al. (18) found a significant association between indoor air pollution and pneumonia.

Variables under sanitation/hygienic factors that were significantly associated with diarrhea at bivariate analysis in this study includes; place of disposal of child's feces, hand washing practices, disposal of household garbage and source of drinking water. At multivariate regression analysis, only place of disposal of child's feces and source of drinking water was significant at 5% (P=0.005 and 0.008 respectively). The Majority of respondents disposed their children's feces in nearby bushes. This inappropriate practice promotes breeding site for flies and other disease agents. As seen from this study, diarrhea was less likely to occur in households with satisfactory disposal of feces (OR=0.512, CI=0.321-0.817).

Oloruntoba, Folarin and Ayede (19) found that lack of proper hand washing after defecating and before or after food preparation by mothers/caregivers predisposes children to diarrhea. Indiscriminate disposal of garbage other than dumpsite was significantly associated with diarrhea occurrence. A study carried out in Uganda by Mbonye (20) and another in West Africa by Sodemann et al. (21) supports this finding. Contaminated water is a major source of diarrheal diseases as established in theories. According to Pruss-Ustun and Corvalan (22) unsafe water and lack of basic sanitation and hygienic practices account for 88% of the disease burden due to diarrhea. Findings from this study showed that the probability of diarrhea occurrence in households with adequate source of drinking water was 0.479 times less likely (OR=0.521, CI=0.322-0.842).Under sanitation/hygienic factors, variables like type of toilet facilities, place of child defecation, frequency in hand washing, disposal of wastewater, buying of food from street vendors and time in getting drinking water was not significantly associated with diarrhea occurrence.

A higher proportion of households had satisfactory place of child defecation compared to 12.2% that were unsatisfactory (defecate outside on the floor). Though this association was statistically insignificant, but noteworthy is that 48.1% of diarrhea outcome was seen in children within households with unsatisfactory place of child defecation compared to 37.7% of those in households with satisfactory place of place of child defecation. Unfortunately, Nigeria recently became the open defecation capital of the world (23).This study found no significant association between frequency of hand washing and diarrhea occurrence, which is supported by the study done by Luby et al. (24) in rural Bangladesh.

Disposal of waste water was found statistically significant in relation to diarrhea as reported by Thiam et al. (25) in their study, but this study had a contrary finding.

Buying of food from food vendors is a predisposing factor to diarrhea as most food vendors lack proper food hygiene and handling practices. Though this study did not find significant association, a study carried out in Northern Vietnam (26) found an association between buying of food from street vendors and childhood diarrhea. Time to obtain drinking water was not significant as the majority of the households used sachet water (defined in this study as adequate source) and since it is sealed, contamination or further contamination with environmental pathogens is less likely.

For variables on breastfeeding/immunization statuses, exclusive breastfeeding in the first six months of life was significantly associated with diarrhea and pneumonia occurrence at the level of bivariate analysis. Findings by Nwaoha, Ohaeri and Amaechi (27) reported that exclusive breastfeeding gave adequate protection against diarrhea. According to the World Health Organization (28), exclusive breastfeeding during the first six months of life reduces the risk of severe or fatal diarrhea, provides the infant with antibodies to wade off infections and many more advantages. Multivariate analysis showed a significant association between exclusive breastfeeding and pneumonia occurrence (P=0.040). This study found that children who were exclusively breastfed were 0.454 times less likely to have pneumonia. As well, Workineh, Haitu and Gultie (29) in a cross sectional study carried out in Southern Ethiopia adduced that, children who were exclusively breastfed were less likely to develop pneumonia.

Conclusion

This study concludes that substandard living conditions contribute to the disease burden and high prevalence of childhood diarrhea and pneumonia in the Ngenevu slum in particular and Nigeria in general. Multivariate regression analysis showed the following factors as independent predictors of diarrhea in children under five years: educational level of mothers/caregivers, number of children under five years living in the households, unsatisfactory place of disposal of child's feces and inadequate source of drinking water. For pneumonia, knowledge of pneumonia, poor ventilation status and exclusive breastfeeding were predictive factors.

This study finding is important as it points to the need for intervention in the housing conditions of these slum dwellers; in provision of portable water and in health education on the importance of high level sanitation and household hygiene. The housing conditions as observed in Ngenevu slum is degrading. It is a fertile environment for epidemic outbreak. Due to non-accessibility of water in the Ngenevu slum, sanitary/hygienic practices were compromised and unsatisfactory. Houses were ill ventilated owing to inadequate number of windows per room and indoor air pollution arising from the use of solid fuels. The practice of exclusive breastfeeding is invaluable in infants considering the immunological content of breast milk and its ability to wade off various infections, but this practice could not be sustained as the majority of the mothers in this low income neighborhood strived to survive and were not readily available (both physically and nutritionally) to attend to their young ones.

The swift implementation of the Integrated Global Action Plan for the Prevention and Control of Diarrhea and Pneumonia (GAPPD), which has exclusive breastfeeding, hand-washing with soap, safe drinking-water and sanitation, reduction of household air pollution as some of its core targets is highly recommended with maximum focus on slums which houses a vast majority of low income settlers. The need also for an inter-sectoral approach to health interventions through the integration of various ministries cannot be over-emphasized.

Limitations

Perceived limitations to this study lies in the case definition of pneumonia which may not be highly specific compared to use of radiological test. The possibility of reporting or recall bias is not ruled out considering the fact that variables were self-reported by mothers/ caregivers. The study was a cross-sectional study hence a cause-effect relationship is difficult to establish. Notwithstanding, this study was able to capture the associations between housing risk factors, diarrhea and pneumonia occurrence in underfive children in the study area.

References

[1] Park K. Textbook of preventive and social medicine, 20th ed.Jabalpur: Banarsidas Bhanot; 2009.

[2] Azeem A. Housing situation in Nigeria. URL:https://www.linkedin.com/pulse/housing/.

[3] Young TK. Population health: Concepts and methods. Oxford: Oxford University Press, 2005.

[4] World Health Organization. Children: Reducing mortality. Geneva: World Health Organization, 2019.URL:https://www.who.int/news-room/fact-sheets/detail/children-reducing/.

[5] United Nations Children's Fund. Childhood disease. URL:https://www.unicef.org/health/childhood-diseases/ .

[6] National Population Commission (NPC) and Inner City Fund (ICF) International. Nigeria Demographic and Health Survey 2013. Abuja, Nigeria. ICF International, 2014.

[7] National Population Commission. Nigeria National Census: Population distribution by sex, state, LGAs and senatorial district 2006. Abuja: National Population Commission, 2006.

[8] Samya V, Stanly AM. Acute diarrhea and acute respiratory infection among less than 5 year old children. A cross sectional study. Int J Sci Stud 2015:3(7):149-53.

[9] Aniwada EC, Oduegwu A, Odoh L, Odonoekuma OE, Ofoegbu FK. Knowledge, perception and misconceptions on family planning among women living in an urban slum in Enugu, Enugu state, Nigeria. Asian J Med Health2017:3(2):1-10.

[10] World Health Organization. Pneumonia key facts, 2016.URL: https://www.who.int/news-room/fact-sheets/detail/pneumonia/.

[11] Chaturvedi M, Roy R, Katiyar K, Agrawal D, Mukherjee S. Forgotten killers of childhood illnesses. Prevalence and practice. Indian J Prev Soc Med 2014:45:110-4.

[12] Nsabimana J, Mureithi C, Habtu M. Factors contributing to diarrhea diseases among children less than five years in Nyanugenge District, Rwanda. J Trop Dis2017;5(2):238. doi:10.4172/2329-891X.1000238.

[13] Yilgwan CS. Okolo SN. Prevalence of diarrhea disease and risk factors in Jos University Teaching Hospital. Nigeria. Ann Afri Med 2012;11:217-21.

[14] Mengistie B, Berhane Y, Worku A. Prevalence of diarrhea and associated risk factors among children under-five years of age in Eastern Ethiopia: A cross-sectional study. Open J Prev Med 2013;3(7):446-53. doi.org/10.4236/ojpm.2013.37060.

[15] Gritly SMO, Elamin MO, Rahimbullah H, Ali AYH, Dhiblaw A, Mohamed EA et al. Risk factors of pneumonia among children under 5 years at a pediatric hospital in Sudan. Int J Med Res Health Sci 2018;7(4):60-8.

[16] Ujunwa FA, Ezeonu CT. Risk factors for acute respiratory tract infections in under five children in Enugu Southeast Nigeria. Am Med Health Sci Res 2014;4(1):95-9.

[17] Fekadu GA, Terefe MW, Aleme GA. Prevalence of pneumonia among under-five children in Este town and the surrounding rural Kebeles, Northwest Ethiopia; a community based cross-sectional study. Sci J Public Health 2014;2(3):150-5. doi:10.11648/j.sjph.20140203.12.

[18] Nirmolia N, Mahanta TG, Bonuah M, Rasaily R, Kotoky RP, Bora R. Prevalence and risk factors of pneumonia in under five children living in slums of Dibrugarh town. Clin Epidemiol Global Health 2018;6:1-4.

[19] Oloruntoba EO, Folarin TB, Ayede AI. Hygiene and sanitation risk factors of diarrheal disease among under-five children in Ibadan, Nigeria. Afr Health Sci2014; 14(4):1001-11.

[20] Mbonye AK. Risk factors for Diarrhea and upper respiratory tract infections among children in a rural area of Uganda. J Health Popul Nutr2004;22(1):52-8.

[21] Sodemann M, Jakobsen MS, Molbak K, Martins C, Aaby P. Episode specific risk factors for progression of acute diarrhea to persistent diarrhea in Western African children. Trans R Soc Tropical Med 1999;93:65-8.

[22] Pruss-Ustun A, Corvalan C. How much burden can be prevented by environmental interventions? Epidemiology 2007;18(1):167-78. doi:10.1097/01.ede.0000239647.26389.80.

[23] Onyedika-ugoeze N. UNICEF says Nigeria leads in global open defecation index. The Guardian 2019 Oct 29.URL: https://guardian.ng/news/unicef

[24] Luby SP, Halder AK, Huda T, Unicomb L, Johnston RB. The effect of hand washing at recommended times with water alone and with soap on child diarrhea in rural Bangledesh: an observational study. PLoS Med 2011;8(6):e1001052.

[25] Thiam S, Diene AN, Funrimann S, Winkler MS, Sy I, Ndione JA et al. Prevalence of diarrhea and risk factors among children under five years old in Mbour, Senegal: A cross-sectional study. Infect Dis Poverty 2017; 6:109. doi:10.1186/s40249-017-0323-1.

[26] Bui VH. The most common causes of and risk factors for diarrhea among children less than five years of age admitted in Dong Anh Hospital, Hanoi. Northern Vietnam. Dissertation. Oslo: University of Oslo, 2006.

[27] Nwaoha AF, Ohaeri CC, Amaechi EC. Prevalence of diarrhea, and associated risk factors, in children aged 0-5 years, at two hospitals in Umuahia, Abia, Nigeria. UNED Res J2017;9(1):7-14.

[28] World Health Organization. Programme of Acute Respiratory Infections & World Health Organization. Malaria Control Unit. (1992). The Overlap in the clinical presentation and treatment of malaria and pneumonia in children: report of a meeting (Geneva, 8 April 1991. World Health Organization. https://apps.who.int/iris/handle/10665/61972

[29] Workineh Y, Haitu D, Gultie T. Determinants of pneumonia among under two children in southern Ethiopia: A case control study of 2016. Curr Pediatr Res 2017;21(4):604-12.

In: Pediatrics and Adolescent Health ISBN: 978-1-68507-490-6
Editors: J. Merrick and M. Morad

Chapter 8

YOUTH MENTAL HEALTH SERVICES IN QATAR

Livia Gilstrap[1], PhD, Muhammad Waqar Azeem[2], MD, Nehdia Hashemi[3], MD and Ahsan Nazeer[2,*], MD

[1]Clinical Psychology, Doha Institute for Graduate Studies, Doha
[2]Department of Psychiatry, Sidra Medicine, Ar-Rayyan, Doha and Weill Cornell Medical College, Doha
[3]Tadawi Medical Center, Doha

ABSTRACT

The last five years have been exciting times for the child and adolescent mental health services (CAMHS) throughout the Middle East and North African region (MENA). Overall in the Middle East, the development of child and adolescent mental health services has lagged behind adult and geriatric psychiatry initiatives. However, during the last decade, numerous initiatives regarding CAMHS have taken place in Qatar. In the current article, we review the history of CAMHS development, the

* Corresponding Author's E-mail: anazeer@sidra.org.

current state of CAMHS facilities, and opportunities for further improvement in the State of Qatar.

INTRODUCTION

Mental health disorders devastate families have a measurable impact on the society and economy of the country (1). Within Qatar, the lifetime prevalence of mental health disorders is estimated to be similar to the rest of the world (2, 3). International and cross-cultural data show that mental health issues are a large part of national health care needs and costs in almost every country (4). Families and societies are disproportionately more affected when it comes to juvenile mental health difficulties since adult caregivers face the responsibility of managing children's treatment (5). From a theoretical standpoint, childhood and adolescence are key stages in the development of mental health disorders since they are the genesis of many of the most prevalent adult mental health problems (6).

QATAR DEMOGRAPHICS

Qatar's population is booming and has doubled in the last three decades. In the 1950s, the population was barely 26,000, rising to 32.7 million in 2019 (7). However, Qatari nationals make up around 12%-15% of the total population. In contrast, the remaining population consists of expats who have called Qatar their home during different phases of their lives (8). Qatar has also witnessed phenomenal economic growth since the 1970s, and most of these expats are the product of a skilled and non-skilled workforce that came from more than eighty-five countries across the world. Because the majority of these people are single male laborers, it is plausible to assume that the population is skewed toward adulthood and that the percentage of children and adolescents in Qatar would be significantly lower than the global average, which, however, is not the case. As per recent estimates, over 25% of the world's population is under

15 (9). As of early 2017, Qatar has around 526,000 children and adolescents under 15, or roughly 22% of the overall population (8).

EPIDEMIOLOGICAL DATA ON YOUTH MENTAL HEALTH

Child and adolescent mental health research is underrepresented globally, but notably in the Middle Eastern countries (10). International literature on youth mental health either reference the region's lack of data (11) or extrapolate the available data to draw assumptions about the region, which does not always paint an accurate picture (12).

This knowledge gap is closing as Middle Eastern countries increasingly emphasize child and adolescent mental health in clinical care, research, and policymaking (13-17). Prevalence data from the available studies appears to be within the normal variation of international estimates of mental disorder prevalence, indicating cross-cultural invariance in mental health.

There is limited data on the prevalence of general mental health diagnoses in representative samples of Qatari youth, while some data exist for particular disorders. For instance, Qatar's youth had a greater overall prevalence of phobias than worldwide estimates (2). Another study examining the prevalence of ADHD in school-aged children in Qatar noted a prevalence rate of 13% (18) compared to a global prevalence of 3.4% -5.29% (19, 20).

In general, clinical and epidemiological research on mental health disorders in Qatar is progressing rapidly; however, the data on children's and adolescents' mental health remains sparse. With only a handful of CAMHS studies, there is insufficient data on child and adolescent mental health to make any summary statements. Some recent studies have noted the prevalence of certain disorders, like autism, in Qatar to be similar to international estimates (21), while others, e.g., the study on phobias (2), have provided compelling evidence that perhaps mental health disorders in youth in this region might present in different proportions than international epidemiological studies of youth mental health. With more highly qualified researchers and clinicians, efforts are underway to develop systematic studies on child and adolescent mental health (22).

As previously noted from the epidemiological studies, the prevalence and type of mental health disorders in these regions are comparable to those observed in other countries (2, 23). As is the case worldwide, about one in every five adults in Qatar is now experiencing a mental health problem, but only one in every four of those experiencing a mental illness is getting mental health care (24). By generalizing the data to the community, we can estimate that around 480,000 individuals in Qatar have a mental illness, but only 120,000 are getting mental health care, leaving a 360,000-person service gap. With population growth that has been constant and rapid, it will take a significant expansion in mental health services to maintain current levels of service provision, much alone erase the above gap. Because the epidemiological data on youth mental health is somewhat lacking, the extent of the service gap for this population is lacking. However, based on the clinical key performance indicators (KPIs), including CAMHS waitlists in outpatient clinics, we know a significant demand exists for CAMHS services in the country.

EXISTING MENTAL HEALTH POLICIES

Qatar established a mental health policy in the 1980s (3, 25). In 2008, with cooperation from the World Health Organization (WHO), the Ministry of Public Health established a National Mental Health Committee. Later, Qatar endorsed and ratified the World Health Organization's Mental Health Action Plan 2013-2020.

Qatar launched its first National Mental Health Strategy (QNMHS) in 2013 with the slogan "Changing minds, changing lives 2013-2018." QNMHS had a considerable influence by increasing the budget for mental health care services, emphasizing community-based care, and establishing training programs for mental health staff (26).

In 2018, under the slogan "Our health, our future," Qatar launched the National Health Strategy 2018-2022 (QNHS), in which "Healthy children and adolescents" were included as one of seven priority populations. "Healthy children and adolescents" does not only focus on children's mental health; instead, it attempts to promote a healthy environment, increased wellbeing, good behaviors, improved nutrition, and establishing a comprehensive national school health program. "Mental health and wellness" was another priority population in QNHS in which the Child and Adolescent Mental Health Services (CAMHS) workstream is responsible for developing CAMHS services throughout the State of Qatar.

MENTAL HEALTH LAW

Qatar's Mental Health Law was formally enacted in November 2016 (25). This legislation outlines fundamental guidelines for providing mental health care to individuals and defines mental health in the Qatari context. The document outlines specific provisions about the rights of mentally ill individuals, including involuntary admission, mandatory community treatment, court-ordered treatment, and sets penalties for medical personnel who violate the fundamental human rights of the individuals with these disorders. The rights of patients to receive treatment in a safe and secure environment that respects their dignity and human rights and the right of patients and their families to give informed consent about their care was also established. Qatar Mental Health law no doubt was a step forward in setting parameters and upholding the fundamental rights of individuals with mental health disabilities; however, it lacked specific guidelines pertaining to child and adolescent mental health, which is needed.

CAMHS IN QATAR: A BRIEF HISTORY

In 2014, there were 13.5 mental health specialists per 100,000 people, less than half the median rate for upper-middle-income nations (26, 27). In 1948, shortly after Hamad Medical Corporation (HMC) opened its door, it admitted its first adult psychiatric patient (28). Hamad Medical Corporation remains the only facility in the country that serves mental health patients of all ages and conditions.

From 1971 to 2015, all child and adolescent mental health treatments at HMC were delivered by doctors trained in adult psychiatry. By 2014, children and adolescents accounted for 23% of mental health outpatient center users (26). In 2015 HMC recruited a child and adolescent psychiatrist and later started expanding its CAMHS services with the addition of psychologists with specialized CAMHS training. The Shafallah Center, founded in 1999, is another institution that was established exclusively to help children and adolescents with developmental disabilities, including cognitive impairment and autism (29).

Historically, school mental health services have always lagged in the country. As of 2017, most individual schools in the country had a nurse, but only a handful had a mental health professional on staff (26). Qatar Council for Healthcare Practitioners (QCHP) started licensing clinicians with bachelor's degrees in psychology to provide mental health treatments inside the school system to cover the above gap.

Along with the above developments, Qatar has developed National Autism Plan and World Innovation Summit for Health (WISH) held an autism conference in Qatar in 2016 (30). As of 2021, Qatar has few child psychiatrists but no inpatient beds for children and adolescents with mental health needs (31).

Hamad Medical Corporation (HMC)

HMC continues to be Qatar's biggest provider of adult and geriatric mental health care. During the last two years, they have also increased the capacity of their CAMHS services by hiring more child and adolescent psychiatrists and psychologists with expertise in dealing with youth. HMC CAMHS accepts most referrals with a few exceptions that include legal matters, incontinence, feeding disorders, domestic violence, and child abuse until child protection procedures are established, and a mental health referral is made. In line with the National Vision and reducing stigma and promoting utilization, the long-term goal is to base Child and Adolescent Psychiatry services at HMC in the community rather than the hospital.

Due to the lack of CAMHS inpatient beds at HMC, youth 13 and younger with severe mental health needs get admitted to either the pediatric hospital section or the adult psychiatric unit. A 24-hour mental health nurse can offer mental health nursing care to these patients on the pediatric unit. Children and adolescents 14 years of age and older are admitted to adult psychiatric inpatient beds. Current growth ambitions include establishing closer ties with hospitals through CAMHS liaisons with emergency departments and establishing specialist CAMHS clinics within hospitals. Additionally, they plan to expand their reach into the community and establish a home care service. Additionally, HMC has launched a child and adolescent psychiatry fellowship program, which recruits one fellow each year for a two-year fellowship. ACGME-I has not accredited the fellowship program till the time of this writing.

Primary Health Care Corporation (PHCC)

PHCC is the primary point of contact for the population's medical and mental health needs. It operates twenty-seven primary health care facilities throughout Qatar. It has recently started piloting programs for mental health services in which physicians detect, assess, and manage mild to moderate mental health disorders. At present, this service is being piloted in a few locations, but plans are to expand the program to the remaining Health Centers. PHCC has also prioritized early detection of autism spectrum disorder (ASD), and all children are being examined at their 18-month well-baby clinic visit. This screening entails the physician at the well-baby clinic completing a questionnaire following an interview with the child's parent or guardian. When an ASD is detected, the child is sent to the Child Rehabilitation Clinic at the Child Development Center at Rumailah Hospital for additional examination, diagnosis, and therapy, if indicated.

SIDRA MEDICINE

Sidra Medicine is a Qatar Foundation initiative that marks a substantial step forward in meeting the State of Qatar's critical health care requirements for women and children (31). The hospital opened its outpatient services in 2016, and the first child and adolescent psychiatry patients were seen in June 2016. CAMHS team consists of psychiatrists and psychologists with support from social work, OT/PT therapists, and speech and language therapists. Services are provided in the outpatient clinic, pediatric emergency department, consultation-liaison service for the medical and surgical floors, and in the pediatrics floor's inpatient psychiatric beds (two modified pediatric beds on pediatric inpatient unit).

CAMHS division at Sidra Medicine aims to promote clinical treatment, research, and education. Their mission is to raise community awareness about youth mental health issues through high-quality clinical services and educational workshops. Children and adolescents aged 5 to 18 years who have a significant emotional problem get treatment. The team specializes in cognitive behavioral therapy, dialectical behavior therapy, narrative therapy, solution-focused therapy, and acceptance commitment therapy. In addition to referrals made by medical professionals, they also accept referrals from teachers or school counselors. Urgent referrals are handled within seven days, while regular referrals are seen within 30 days.

Sidra Medicine's CAMHS consultation-liaison program is the Middle East's first comprehensive psychiatric consultation for children and adolescents. Around 18-20% of medical inpatient hospitalizations contain a mental health component. If the care is not provided on time, it results in a longer hospital stay, increased hospital costs, a greater number of surgeries, and an increased rate of re-hospitalizations. It has been demonstrated that early participation of CAMHS improves clinical results by improving patient treatment, staff satisfaction, comfort, and engagement. Consultation services include evaluation and treatment recommendations for complex co-occurring medical and psychiatric disorders such as mood disorders, suicidal or self-injurious thoughts, behavioral problems, medical illnesses associated with psychiatric disorders, chronic pain, failure to thrive, adjustment to chronic medical illnesses, and organic neuropsychiatric syndromes.

Numerous grant-funded programs focusing on Qatari youth are also underway. Currently funded research includes assessing the validity of and developing normative data for Arab speaking adolescents on standard psychological measures, parenting variables and mental health, the neurogenomics of ADHD and ASD, mental health outcomes for specific medical conditions, infant mental health in relation to postpartum depression, and psychotic experiences.

Additionally, the division provides instructional services to various higher education institutions, including Weil Cornell Medical School-Qatar, Doha Institute for Graduate Studies, and Qatar University.

Sidra Medicine's Child Abuse and Neglect Services (S-CAP)

Data on child abuse and neglect in Qatar is limited; nonetheless, informal polls indicate that child abuse is an area of concern. As per the Ministry of Development Planning and Statistics, June 2015 report, the Protection and Social Rehabilitation Center (AMAN) have recorded 145 child abuse instances in 2007 and 853 in 2012. Between 2009 and 2016, the pediatric emergency center in Al Sadd has also recorded 126 such incidents.

Qatar's legislation on child protection (Law No. 11 of 2004, Article 269) states, "Whoever jeopardizes a person under sixteen or a person incapable of protecting himself due to his mental, psychological or health conditions shall be punished with imprisonment for a term not exceeding two years and a fine not exceeding ten thousand Qatari Riyals (QAR 10.000). The penalty shall be up to three years in prison and a fine up to fifteen thousand Qatari Riyals (QAR 15.000), if the person is left alone in a deserted place or if the guardian is the offender" (32). In 1995, Qatar ratified the Convention on the Rights of the Child (33) and is working on enhancing its legislation to bring it up to international standards by developing new laws and updating current ones. Child rights protection is a priority in accordance with Qatar's strategic development plan, Qatar National Vision 2030. (34, 35).

The Sidra Child Advocacy Program (S-CAP) establishment demonstrates the country's continued commitment to child rights protection. The S-CAP team provides 24-hour telephone assistance to healthcare experts throughout Qatar and coordinates medical assessments, investigations, and follow-up for child abuse victims. It collaborates closely with other elements of the country's multidisciplinary team, including the Police and Public Prosecution, Forensic Medicine physicians hired by the Ministry of the Interior, the Protection and Social Rehabilitation Center (AMAN), and the Family Consultation Center. Child abuse prevention activities include educating healthcare personnel in the community and conducting media campaigns to raise public awareness about child safety. S-CAP created a dedicated Child Advocacy Helpline for young people and members of the public to call in the event of child abuse or suspicion of child abuse.

Naufar Center for the Treatment of Substance Abuse

The Naufar is a specialized program that opened its doors to treat substance use disorders in youth 12 to 18. Their team consists of a child and adolescent psychiatrist, an internist, a family therapist, an occupational therapist, a social worker, an exercise physiologist and physiotherapist, an art psychotherapist.

Their inclusion criteria include adolescents who exhibit problematic substance use ranging from recreational to pathological and adolescents who exhibit co-occurring disorders such as ADHD, anxiety disorders, mood disorders, conduct disorders, and behavioral disorders associated with substance experimentation. Youth with significant mental health needs, including active psychosis, suicidal ideation, or reported suicidal plan, or significant suicidal ideation or incident history; considerable risk to self or others, or considerable history of property damage; and youth with moderate to significant special educational needs are excluded.

Community resources

As mentioned above, numerous community-based organizations provide CAMHS-related services to a specific population or disorder (e.g., cognitive impairment and autism – Shafallah Center, family violence – Aman Protection and Social Rehabilitation Center, substance use – Naufar). Additionally, community groups focus on public awareness (e.g., Weyak Mental Health Friends Association) and organizations that provide some forms of CAMHS primary screening (e.g., Wifaq Family Consulting Center currently offers some types of developmental consultations). Only the Shafallah Center is exclusively focused on children and adolescents (29). Along with the above, numerous private centers offer mental health services to children and adolescents. MIND Institute is among the largest and has an array of comprehensive mental health services, including recently established vocational opportunities for the youth who qualify their criteria.

FUTURE OF CAMHS LANDSCAPE

This section identifies three critical areas for future growth in CAMHS.

A chronic shortage of CAMHS inpatient beds exists in numerous countries across the globe (36, 37). The similar is the case in Qatar, where there is a significant need for a dedicated child and adolescent psychiatry inpatient unit. The risks of placing youth with adults in inpatient institutions are many and possibly self-evident. Apart from the risks, the particular requirements of CAMHS patients in these settings are also unique and can not be met in an adult psychiatric inpatient setting. The present workarounds (e.g., utilizing pediatric beds in Sidra Medicine) are currently insufficient to meet the demands. This issue, however, is not likely to be resolved soon, but some positive steps are underway.

Mental health training programs in child and adolescent psychiatry and clinical psychology are a relatively recent development in Qatar. Both Sidra Medicine and HMC have fellowship programs in child and adolescent psychiatry. The American College of Graduate Medical Education-International (ACGME-I) has accredited Sidra Medicine's curriculum, making it the first in the world to get that accreditation. The Doha Institute for Graduate Studies' new MSc in Clinical Psychology includes a semester-long practicum at Sidra Medicine but does not provide a formal CAMHS focus. However, there is still a need for specialized CAMHS training programs in allied disciplines such as nursing and social work. Additionally, training should be targeted towards Qataris and nationals of adjacent countries since these individuals are more likely to remain in the region and help local communities after completing their studies.

We require epidemiological data on illness prevalence and demographic characteristics to make evidence-based decisions and policies. While there are some parallels in mental health across cultures, there is sufficient evidence of cross-cultural heterogeneity to make the absence of child and adolescent mental health data from Qatar a significant gap. Arab children and adolescents are underrepresented in worldwide data sets and models of youth mental health. Due to a lack of data from the region, the prevalence of various disorders in children and adolescents is unknown. The causal models used have unclear relationships to disorder development, and the unique characteristic patterns of Arab families, particularly Qatari families, are not examined concerning youth mental health.

Aligning evidence and policy leads to more targeted intervention and policy development, more efficient economic asset allocation, and more effective use of community resources.

CONCLUSION

This is a moment of rapid growth in society, with development and progress occurring in practically every field. Not all systems have advanced equally as a result of the expansion. While some systems and initiatives are cutting-edge, others have been imagined and planned but have yet to gain traction. For CAMHS services, the last decade has been challenging, but numerous positive strides have been made during the previous five years. If this trajectory continues, there will be a reason to be optimistic about the future of the mental health care of youth and families.

References

[1] Bener A, Zirie MA, Kim E-J, Al Buz R, Zaza M, Al-Nufal M, et al. Measuring burden of diseases in a rapidly developing economy: state of Qatar. Glob J Health Sci 2012;5(2):134-44.

[2] Bener A, Ghuloum S, Dafeeah EE. Prevalence of common phobias and their socio-demographic correlates in children and adolescents in a traditional developing society. Afr J Psychiatry 2011;14(2):140-5.

[3] Ghuloum S, Ibrahim MA. Psychiatry in Qatar. Int Psychiatry 2006;3(4):16-8.

[4] Murray CJ, Vos T, Lozano R, Naghavi M, Flaxman AD, Michaud C, et al. Disability-adjusted life years (DALYs) for 291 diseases and injuries in 21 regions, 1990–2010: a systematic analysis for the Global Burden of Disease Study 2010. Lancet 2012;380(9859):2197-223.

[5] Kheir N, Ghoneim O, Sandridge AL, Al-Ismail M, Hayder S, Al-Rawi F. Quality of life of caregivers of children with autism in Qatar. Autism 2012;16(3):293-8.

[6] Rutter M, Kim-Cohen J, Maughan B. Continuities and discontinuities in psychopathology between childhood and adult life. J Child Psychol Psychiatry 2006;47(3-4):276-95.

[7] Authority PaS. Monthly figures on total population 2019. URL: https://www.psa.gov.qa/en/statistics1/StatisticsSite/pages/population.aspx.

[8] Statistics MoDPa. Qatar in figures 2017. URL: https://www.psa.gov.qa/en/statistics/Statistical%20Releases/General/QIF/Qatar_in_Figures_32_2017_EN.pdf.

[9] Bank TW. Population ages 0-14 (% of total population) 2019. URL: https://data.worldbank.org/indicator/SP.POP.0014.TO.ZS.

[10] Gater R, Saeed K. Scaling up action for mental health in the Eastern Mediterranean Region: an overview. East Mediterr Health J 2015;12(7):535-45.

[11] Obermeyer CM, Bott S, Sassine AJ. Arab adolescents: Health, gender, and social context. J Adolesc Health 2015;57(3):252-62.

[12] Whiteford HA, Degenhardt L, Rehm J, Baxter AJ, Ferrari AJ, Erskine HE, et al. Global burden of disease attributable to mental and substance use disorders: findings from the Global Burden of Disease Study 2010. Lancet. 2013;382(9904):1575-86.

[13] Al Riyami AA, Al Adawi SH, Al Kharusi HA, Morsi MM, Jaju SS. Health services utilization by school going Omani adolescents and youths with DSM IV mental disorders and barriers to service use. Int J Ment Health Syst 2009;3(1):22.

[14] Jaju S, Al-Adawi S, Al-Kharusi H, Morsi M, Al-Riyami A. Prevalence and age-of-onset distributions of DSM IV mental disorders and their severity among school going Omani adolescents and youths: WMH-CIDI findings. Child Adolesc Psychiatry Ment Health 2009;3(1):29.

[15] Mahfouz AA, Al-Gelban KS, Al Amri H, Khan MY, Abdelmoneim I, Daffalla AA, et al. Adolescents' mental health in Abha City, Southwestern Saudi Arabia. Int J Psychiatr Med 2009;39(2):169-77.

[16] Mahfoud Z, Abdulrahim S, Taha MB, Harpham T, El Hajj T, Makhoul J, et al. Validation of the Arab Youth Mental Health scale as a screening tool for depression/anxiety in Lebanese children. Child Adolesc Psychiatry Ment Health 2011;5:9.

[17] Alyahri A, Goodman R. Validation of the Arabic strengths and difficulties questionnaire and the development and well-being assessment. East Mediterr Health J 2006;12(suppl 2):S138-46.

[18] Bradshaw LG, Kamal M. Prevalence of ADHD in Qatari school-age children. J Attent Disord. 2016;21(5):442-9.

[19] Polanczyk G, de Lima MS, Horta BL, Biederman J, Rohde LA. The worldwide prevalence of ADHD: A systematic review and metaregression analysis. Am J Psychiatry 2007;164(6):942-8.

[20] Polanczyk GV, Salum GA, Sugaya LS, Caye A, Rohde LA. Annual research review: A meta-analysis of the worldwide prevalence of mental disorders in children and adolescents. J Child Psychol Psychiatry 2015;56(3):345-65.

[21] Alshaban F, Aldosari M, Al-Shammari H, El-Hag S, Ghazal I, Tolefat M, et al. Prevalence and correlates of autism spectrum disorder in Qatar: a national study. J Child Psychol Psychiatry Allied Discipl 2019;60(12):1254-68.

[22] Gilstrap LL, Nazeer A, Azeem MW, Archard R, Ather M. Family characteristics, parenting styles, and youth mental health in Qatar. Doha: International Family Institute/Qatar Foundation, Qatar National Research Fund (QNRF), 2019.

[23] Bener A, Ghuloum S, Dafeeah EE, Al-Yazidi T, Mustapha A, Zakareia A. Lifetime prevalence of common mental disorders in Qatar: Using WHO composite international diagnostic interview (WHO-CIDI). Int J Clin Psychiatr Ment Health 2014;2(1):38-46.

[24] Zolezzi M, Abdulrhim S, Isleem N, Zahrah F, Eltorki Y. Medical comorbidities in patients with serious mental illness: a retrospective study of mental health patients attending an outpatient clinic in Qatar. Neuropsychiatr Dis Treat2017;13:2411-8.

[25] Abou-Saleh MT, Ibrahim MA. Mental health law in Qatar. Int Psychiatry 2013;10(4):88-90.

[26] Sharkey T. Mental health strategy and impact evaluation in Qatar. B J Psychiatr Int 2017;14(1):18-21.

[27] Okasha A, Karam E, Okasha T. Mental health services in the Arab world. World Psychiatry 2012;11(1):52-4.

[28] Kronfol Z, Ghuloum S, Weber A. Country in focus: Qatar. Asian J Psychiatry 2013;6(3):275-7.

[29] Shafallah. About Shafallah 2020 URL: http://www.shafallah.org.qa/En/Pages/AboutShafallah.aspx.

[30] Munir KM, Lavelle TA, Helm DT, Rustamov I, Azeem W. Developing countries and autism. Encyclopedia of autism spectrum disorders. New York: Springer, 2017:1-10.

[31] Waqar Azeem M. Child and adolescent mental health services in Qatar: Past, present, and future. J Am Acad Child Adolesc Psychiatry 2017;56(10):S84.

[32] Qatar Penal Code. Exposing Children to Danger, 268 Article, 2004.

[33] Commissioner UNHROotH. Qatar 2019 URL: https://www.ohchr.org/EN/Countries/MENARegion/Pages/QAIndex.aspx.

[34] Planning GSfD. Qatar National Vision 2030, 2008. URL: https://www.psa.gov.qa/en/qnv1/pages/default.aspx.

[35] Statistics MoDPa. Realising Qatar National Vision 2030. The Right to development June 2015. URL: https://www.psa.gov.qa/en/knowledge/Doc/HDR/Qatar_Fourth_National_HDR_Realising_QNV2030_The_Right_to_Development_2015_EN.pdf.

[36] Hazen EP, Prager LM. A quiet crisis: pediatric patients waiting for inpatient psychiatric care. J Am Acad Child Adolesc Psychiatry 2017;56(8):631-3.

[37] Morris J, Belfer M, Daniels A, Flisher A, Villé L, Lora A, et al. Treated prevalence of and mental health services received by children and adolescents in 42 low-and-middle-income countries. J Child Psychol Psychiatry 2011;52(12):1239-46.

SECTION TWO: ADOLESCENT HEALTH

In: Pediatrics and Adolescent Health ISBN: 978-1-68507-490-6
Editors: J. Merrick and M. Morad

Chapter 9

PERCEIVED ACHIEVEMENT OF SUBJECT LEARNING OUTCOMES, PEDAGOGICAL STRATEGY, FACILITATING SKILLS AND ACADEMIC PERFORMANCE OF UNIVERSITY ENGINEERING STUDENTS

Rodney Wai-Chi Chu[1,*], PhD,
Daniel TL Shek[1], PhD, Alex Ying-yin Wong[2], PhD
and Ming-yin Chan[2], PhD
[1]Department of Applied Social Sciences,
The Hong Kong Polytechnic University, Hong Kong, PR China
[2]Department of Building Services Engineering,
The Hong Kong Polytechnic University, Hong Kong, PR China

* Corresponding Author's E-mail: rodney.chu@polyu.edu.hk.

ABSTRACT

Based on students' responses, this study examined the inter-relationships amongst perceived achievement of learning outcomes, teacher's pedagogical strategy as well as facilitating skills, and professional knowledge of the students. Pre-test and post-test data on the achievement of learning outcomes (N=36) and data based on additional questions in the post questionnaire addressing pedagogical strategies and facilitating skills of the teachers were collected. Results showed that after flipped classroom learning, posttest scores on the subject intended learning outcomes were higher than the pretest scores. Pearson correlation analyses also showed that perceived achievement of the intended learning outcomes of the subject and teachers' pedagogical knowledge/strategies as well as facilitating skills were positively correlated with academic performance of students.

INTRODUCTION

In this chapter we study a one-year subject program offered by the Department of Building Services Engineering of The Hong Kong Polytechnic University, attempting to examine whether students' learning is facilitated through flipped classroom teaching and learning. The inter-relationships amongst students' perceived achievement of learning outcomes, the teachers' pedagogical strategy and facilitating skills, and academic performance, were examined. The subject under study was entitled "Light, man and environment" [BSE1D02], which is one of the introductory courses offered in the first semester for those first-year engineering students belonging to a four-year program of the department. In psychology, perception is the process of becoming aware of something, including evaluation and judgment about others (1, 2), which is experiencing stimuli through our senses. What we have received and learnt to our memory depends on the perception. As such, our perception and learning process may also be affected by what we have learnt (2). A study by Glover et al. (3) showed that what we have learnt from experience affects our perception significantly. It is somewhat like 'apperception', which is defined by Merriam-Webster Dictionary as 'mental perception'; it is another way for us to receive message or information occurs through integrating of our experience and what we have learnt, especially the process of "learning or understanding" perceived in terms of their experience. Simply, what we have received or learnt (stimuli or perceptions) will be used for comparison and be related to the information we collected in the past. As William James in 1890 (4) stated,

> "Apperception is an extremely useful word in pedagogics, which offers a convenient name for a process to which every teacher must frequently refer. But it verily means nothing more than the act of taking a thing into the mind. The key of perception is that every impression that comes in from without – be it a sentence which we hear, an object of vision, or an effluvium which assails our nose – no sooner will enter our consciousness and make connection with the other materials already there, and finally producing what we call our reaction. The connections it strikes into are determined by our past experiences and the 'associations' of the present sort of impression with them."

As described by Adedowura and Tayo, "perception is the reaction elicited when an impression is perceived from without after making connection with other materials in the consciousness (memory)" (p.165). Reaction triggered is dependent on perception on prior knowledge. This view also aligns with the study of Glover et al. (3) that background knowledge affects perception. As a result, students' perception of the achievement of the subject learning outcomes, pedagogical knowledge, and facilitating skills are dependent on what and how information (i.e., indicative syllabus and pedagogical strategy) has been delivered/transferred by the teachers. More specifically, the expected learning outcomes to be achieved by the students are dependent on what have been taught (i.e., indicative syllabus) by the teacher.

In addition, perception may also be influenced by our experience, sensation, levels of interest and attention, as well as ways of interpretation (2). Shulman (5) categorized teacher knowledge into different categories. One of the categories focuses on the concept of "pedagogical content knowledge," which integrates the details of a specific subject and the knowledge for teaching of that subject. This concept of pedagogical content knowledge is the most basic ingredient of teachers' knowledge and has been studied widely in the scientific literature (6). Research findings have shown that there is a significant relationship between teacher's knowledge and their instructions (7). Hence, to enhance the effectiveness of teaching, teachers not only need to understand the subject content thoroughly, but also need to utilize pedagogical strategies to escalate students' engagement through collaborative tasks in the classroom. Adedowura and Tayo (2) stated that how students perceive the subject knowledge gained from the teacher may significantly affect students' academic performance. As abovementioned, the combination of content and pedagogy are useful for teachers to enhance student learning. Therefore, subject teacher's knowledge should know exactly what concepts and knowledge can be transferred. If a teacher wants his/her students to learn and understand the flipped learning approach, one has to have the related knowledge – this refers to one's knowledge of subject content and pedagogy – for teaching it. Then, based on teacher's professional knowledge, one can explain the content and instruction that would be used before and during class time. For instance, students can experience what it is like to undertake the flipped learning approach. They will be more likely to understand the ways and find it engaging and interactive.

During the past few decades, e-learning technology provides different ways to support online learning and teaching contexts in higher education programs. Active and collaborative learning integrated with online learning, a kind of blended learning model, provides a better learning alternative for students as compared to rely solely on the conventional face-to-face classroom-based learning. The flipped classroom is a common form of blended-learning model which incorporates classroom and online learning experiences (8, 9). Through this blended learning approach, students acquire basic knowledge or relevant concepts via an online learning management platform prior to class; then, they "work through problems, advance concepts, and engage in collaborative learning" in the classroom (10, 11). This strategy shifts from teacher-centeredness to student-centeredness and highlights the importance of self-regulated learning and motivation for intrinsic reasons that are associated with effictive learning of knowledge.

A meta-analysis study (12) showed that blended learning provides an effective means to teaching and learning in comparison with the traditional face-to-face approach or online learning mode. Research has shown that the flipped classroom promotes positive student outcomes. For example, McLaughlin et al. (13) reported that examination performance and commitment of students improved in a flipped pharmaceutics course. Piere and Fox (14) also reported the enhanced performance and perception of students in a flipped renal pharmacotherapy module. Blended-learning was also associated with better student learning outcomes in different health-related programs (15-17).

The role of professional educators (e.g., subject teachers) in the flipped classroom is very crucial and often more demanding than that in traditional classroom practice. During class time, they need to observe and assess the work of their students and provide the students appropriate feedback. They need to reflect on their practice, improve the instruction, and manage chaos in the classroom when it happens. Apart from these challenges, they are expected to design flipped activities that are meaningful to students, and they must provide incentive and grab the attention of students in both in- and out-of-class activities. As there are local and international students with diverse background/culture or disciplines taking the foundation subjects at university level, it is imperative for the subject teacher to design the active learning curriculum component for these students, make the course more interesting, and provide them with more engagement in class.

Having said all these, one of the key issues need to be addressed is how to give students the best possible collaboration, co-operation, and peer interaction experience by adopting student-centered approaches, in a way that is cost-effective for staff members. Therefore, the subject teacher has the responsibility to provide more learning opportunities for students who can then enter their professionals equipped to function in a collaborative context. In view of this, the flipped classroom approach provides opportunities for students to be prepared before coming to class, thereby giving direct interaction among students through meaningful group activities (18).

To engage in a flipped classroom approach, four basic elements of flipped learning that are developed from Flipped Learning Network in 2014, which known as the Four Pillars of FLIP (19), are involved in teaching practice. This pedagogical approach creates interactive learning environments in which the educators able to provide appropriate guidance for students while applying theories concepts, integrating different areas of knowledge, and having creative engagement with the students. These elements are described below.

- Flexible environment: with the use of online educational technologies delivering course materials outside the classroom, this would free up in-class time for having active and collaborative learning activities and to promote support from classmates and teachers. In this study, with the application of flipped-learning model, an e-learning management system was developed for the selected subject – "Light, Man and Environment" (BSE1D02). This is a competency-based course which includes learning resources and online quizzes. The online platform was designed in such a way which enabled students to learn independently at their free time at own pace, and shift the learning responsibility from the facilitator to the learner. Through this process, self-directed learning direction and paces can be promoted.
- Learning culture: using classroom time to deepen students' knowledge and enrich their learning experience through active participation of group discussions and activities.
- Intentional content: Educational material is intentionally used to maximize conventional face-to-face lecture hours for employing

student-centred and active learning strategies, depending on the level of the students and subject matter.

- Professional educator/subject teacher: professional educator/ subject teacher takes the role of facilitator who normally possesses basic teaching/facilitating skills for teaching and learning (20, 21), where "teaching is a process of continuous personal development and professional self-discovery alongside an emerging understanding of the teaching and learning process" (2). Barrows and Tamblyn (22) also argued that the facilitator is the key, who will assist students to think more deeply and critically. Hence, the facilitator in the classroom activities should not dominate the activities of the learners; rather, the facilitator should promote peer-learning group, monitor learners' learning progress, encourage active group discussion from team members and step in where necessary, to enhance student learning in the classroom (23-26). One can also grant the learners more time to develop their creativity and innovation. In addition, the learners should also engage in interactive discussion and role play so that the process of learning become all around. Eggen and Kauchak (27) emphasized that integration and interaction skills are crucial for teaching and learning.

In this study, we examined how the perceived achievement of learning outcomes and the teaching and learning process are related to the academic performance of the students. In fact, some personality factors including anxiety, motivation, achievement, and level of interest have effects on students' academic performance (28). A study by Ford (29) also showed that personality factor of students such as high self-efficacy could make them performed better than those with low self-efficacy. Similarly, students may perform poorly when having lower self-concept. As described by Adediwura and Tayo (2), teacher variables such as teachers' knowledge of the subject matter, teaching skills, and teaching experiences were related to student academic performance.

To further understand the relationships among teacher's knowledge of the students' understanding, pedagogical strategies, facilitating skills, and academic performance of students, we adopted Allport's (1) psychological concept of perception as "the way through which we evaluate people we are familiar with" (30). Allport reasoned that in person perception, the perceiver is the "judge" and person perceived the 'other'. The above concept and approach have been adopted by Adediwura and Tayo (2). Therefore, the engineering students served as judges in evaluating the knowledge received, pedagogical strategies, and facilitating skills used by the teacher. Generally speaking, we tested the following hypotheses:

- Hypothesis 1: There would be positive changes in the students' responses to items assessing the subject intended learning outcomes.
- Hypothesis 2: There would be a positive relationship between students' perception of achievement of the subject learning outcomes and students' academic performance.
- Hypothesis 3: There would be a positive relationship between students' perception of teachers' pedagogical knowledge/strategy and students' academic performance.
- Hypothesis 4: There would be a positive relationship between students' perception of teachers' facilitating skills and students' academic performance.

In a nutshell, the focus of this research is to analyze first-year engineering students' perceptions of different aspects of a subject (including achievement of subject learning outcomes, teachers' pedagogical knowledge/strategies, and teachers' facilitating skills) and their outcome performance. Besides, whether students' flipped classroom would help to achieve the learning outcomes would also be explored.

OUR STUDY

A one-group pre- and post-test design was adopted in the study. A total of 57 full-time undergraduate engineering students were invited to participate in this study. In the end, 36 students were successfully matched.

This foundation course ("Light, man and environment" [BSE1D02]), which was implemented in the 1st semester of 2016, was redesigned according to the aforementioned flipped learning model (Flipped Learning). In the first semester of 2017/18, selected lectures of the subject adopted the flipped classroom pedagogy. Bloom's idea of taxonomy (31) was applied to the flipped classroom in order to facilitate student learning at understanding level before they got into the specific lecture, whereas student learning would be deepened at application/synthesis level by adopting collaborative learning which enabled them to have more hands-on experience in class time. For example, students were assigned out-of-class learning activities at least one or two weeks before they attended the lecture. The series of out-of-class activities included watching relevant videos (e.g., YouTube) and answering a set of multiple-choice questions covering the following five topics - human vision and interaction of light with matter, light and colour: basic terminology, daylight and artificial light sources, photometric characteristics of light sources, and light and health. This series of activities aimed to strengthen students' understanding of relevant definitions, concepts, and theories before coming to lectures, and help them reflect their learning at understanding level.

Before starting the in-class activities (e.g., jigsaw or group work), students were pre-assigned to a 5-person or 6-person groups and one student in each group served as the group leader. Stand-alone segments on 1) Lamp Filament, 2) Lamp Fluorescent, 3) Lamp HID, and 4) Lamp LED were divided by the subject teacher who subsequently assigned each student in the jigsaw group to focus on one segment. According to Social Psychology Network 2019 (32), students were given time to go over their pre-assigned topics/sections in order to get familiar with them. Afterward, the subject teacher formed 'expert groups' by inviting one student from each jigsaw group to work on the same topics/sections. In these groups, students discussed the main points of their topics/sections and made a presentation based on the jigsaw group discussion. Finally, students re-joined their jigsaw groups to present their topics/sections to the group. The subject teacher/facilitator addressed the key point and reinforced the concepts of the topics with students to deepen students' understanding about the content (i.e., reflection and refraction) and how these could expand and create their intellectual capacity beyond disciplinary domains. Appropriate intervention would be made by the subject teacher/facilitator if any group encountered difficulties. The above jigsaw technique, which was designed by social psychologist Elliot Aronson in 1971 (33), was meant to "promote better learning, improve student motivation, increases enjoyment of the learning experience" (p.59). The effectiveness of student learning could be evaluated from their case study seminars, presentations (or quizzes), and examination by the end of semester, which were the three major assessment items of the subject.

Pretest and posttest measures in the form of questionnaires were used to assess students' perception of their learning experience on the flipped classroom using five-point Likert scales, with response options ranging from 'strongly agree' to 'strongly disagree'. The questionnaire in this study was based on the instruments used by McNaught et al. (34), McLuckie and Topping (10), and Pintrich et al. (35). The questionnaire was divided into four sections. In Section A, there are five subject learning outcome items which are identical in the pretest and posttest questionnaire. They were designed to understand students' perception of their achievement towards the intended subject learning outcomes (ISLOs). The posttest questionnaire contains items assessed student learning experiences of flipped classroom. For instance, Section B contains nine items about teaching and learning environment. In Section C, there are eight items about the usefulness and applicability of the learning materials. Finally, Section D contains eight items assessing facilitators' facilitating skills and one open-ended question measuring the general comments and/or feedback of the students. Pre and post surveys to evaluate their flipped classroom experience, one after the commencement of the flipped learning approach and another after the completion of the flipped learning activities in the classroom, were done subject to anonymous voluntary participation by the students. Because of the anonymous nature in doing the surveys, their responses to the questions would have no association to the final grade of the participating students of this subject.

FINDINGS

Regarding internal consistency of the measures, Cronbach's α of the instrument for each subscale ranged between 0.674 and 0.845 (see Table 1), and the Cronbach's α for the total scale was 0.951, showing very good reliability.

A total of 36 match-paired sample of engineering students participated in the study. A paired sample t-test with α 0.05 was used to compare students' pre- and post-test responses based on their perception of the subject learning outcomes (see Table 2). As predicted, Table 2 shows that post-test mean scores were significantly higher than the pre-test mean scores. The greatest increase in terms of students' perception of the achievement of the learning outcomes are a) the ability to discuss the impact of artificial lighting on people and the environment, b) the ability to illustrate the interrelationship between light, human, and the environment, and c) the ability to give an account of the importance of light in their daily life. Such significant changes in the post scores imply that the subject teacher had a significant contribution and impact on the students in terms of the transferring knowledge of the topics and implementing pedagogical strategies. The findings basically supported hypothesis 1.

Table 1. Constructs, subscales, items and Cronbach's α coefficients of the flipped learning instrument

Constructs	Subscales	No. of items	Reliability
Teaching and Learning environment	Active learning	2	.786
	Teaching for understanding	3	.808
	Workload	2	.814
	Relationship with other students	2	.839
Usefulness and applicability of the learning materials	Motivation	4	.732
	Self-directed learning	2	.674
	Integrated learning	2	.749
Facilitator's facilitating skills	Basics	3	.776
	Helping by Talking	3	.834
	Winding up	2	.845
Total scales		25	.951

To understand the relationship between students' perceived achievement of the SILOs and their academic performance (e.g., presentation, report, seminar, and overall grade), Pearson correlation analyses were used. Results showed a significant and positive correlation between students' perception of achievement of the subject learning outcome(s) (ILO1) and their academic performance with Pearson moment correlation values - presentation ($r = 0.38$, $p < 0.05$) and seminar ($r = 0.36$, $p < 0.05$) (see Table 3). Apparently, students' academic performance was related to their perceived achievement of the learning outcome(s).

Besides, Pearson correlation analyses showed a significant positive correlation between sub-scales of flipped classroom including workload ($r = 0.331$, $p < 0.05$), relationship with other students ($r = 0.424$, $p < 0.05$); ($r = 0.545$, $p < 0.05$), winding up ($r = 0.349$, $p < 0.05$), and students' academic performance (Table 4). Linkage was also found between presentation and seminar results and the sub-scale of "relationship with other students." The subscale comprises of underlying components "felt the sense of belonging to my group when taking part of jigsaw collaborative activities," and "had fruitful discussion with others in my group when taking part of jigsaw collaborative activities." This result implies that there is a significant and positive relationship between collaborative learning designed for the students and the students' assessment results or performance. Table 4 also shows that the sub-scale pedagogy, 'Workload' – which comprises of underlying components including "reasonable amount of time spent on flipped classroom" and "reasonable amount of work was assigned" – was positively and significantly correlated with students' academic performance.

Table 2. Results of paired sample t-test on responses of the achievement of the subject learning outcomes (SILOs) (N = 36)

	Pre		**Post**				
	M	*SD*	*M*	*SD*	*d.f.*	*t*	*P*
ILO1). I can give an account of the importance of light in their daily life.	3.64	.833	3.89	.622	35	-2.049	.048*
ILO2). I can describe the nature of light and compare the properties of natural and artificial light sources.	3.61	.803	3.78	.591	35	-1.099	.279
ILO3). I can illustrate the interrelationship between light, human and the environment.	3.56	.809	3.89	.398	35	-2.646	.012*
ILO4). I can explain the requirements of lighting to satisfy human biological, psychological and physiological needs.	3.50	.941	3.78	.540	35	-1.616	.115
ILO5). I can discuss the impact of artificial lighting on people and the environment.	3.25	.906	3.69	.710	35	-2.935	.006**

Note *p<.05, **p<.01, ***p<.001.

Table 3. Correlations, means, and standard deviations of study variables [Subject learning outcomes vs academic performance (e.g., presentation and seminar)]

	Mean	s.d.	1	2	3
1. Presentation	2.77	0.46	1		
2. Seminar	2.72	0.37	.814**	1	
3. ILO1	2.12	0.82	.380*	.360*	1

Note *p<.05, **p<.01, ***p<.001.

Table 4. Correlations, means, and standard deviations of study variables (sub-scale of pedagogy vs academic performance)

	Mean	s.d.	1	2	3	4	5	6	7
1. Overall grade	3.36	0.43	1						
2. Presentation	3.19	0.58	.038	1					
3. Report	3.25	0.47	-.021	.158	1				
4. Seminar	3.22	0.40	.015	.814**	.702**	1			
5. Workload	3.76	0.67	.331*	.214	-.147	.068	1		
6. Relationship with other students	3.71	0.73	.199	.545**	.052	.424*	.511**	1	
7. Winding Up	3.90	0.48	.349*	.312	-.141	.134	.566**	.404*	1

Note *p<.05, **p<.01, ***p<.001.

Furthermore, Pearson correlation analyses showed that there was a positive significant relationship between students' perception of teachers' facilitating skills (Winding up) – namely, "The facilitator had good time control during the lecture," and "The facilitator discussed the usefulness of this flipped classroom pedagogy with us," with academic performance of the students (e.g., overall grade). Results also showed the significant relationship between students' experience of flipped learning (e.g., workload and relationship with other students) and academic performance (e.g., overall grade, presentation, and seminar). During jigsaw collaborative activities, students worked collaboratively with their team members to solve group-based activities during the classroom (36). Students not only gained support and knowledge from the subject teacher as a facilitator during the active learning activities, but also developed their generic skills such as problem-solving and communication with other team members. In short, the findings supported hypotheses 2, 3, and 4.

CONCLUSION

The paired sample t-test results showed significant differences in terms of students' subject intended learning outcomes after the intervention of the flipped approach. It is indicated that enhancements might have been made due to the flipped classroom integrating online learning, collaborative and cooperative learning activities, tailor-made subject content, and teachers' professional guidance and input. As for subject learning outcomes, participating students are able to explain, describe, and discuss relevant subject ILOs according to different levels of Bloom Taxonomy. The participating students agree that what they have learnt and gained or the teaching and learning strategies used by the subject teacher or facilitator might be able to enhance their outcomes in educational contexts. Moreover, online learning management system and in-class collaborative activities both can help to integrate different outcomes/results and construct knowledge relevant to different educational contexts. The findings are also consistent with previous studies highlighting the value of flipped classroom teaching.

Table 2 shows a statistically significant improvement in students' post-survey scores of the subject intended learning outcomes (e.g., ILO1, ILO3, and ILO5) after the intervention of flipped classroom, supporting Hypothesis 1. This finding is consistent with the findings of former studies where flipped classroom approach in education yields a significant change in student learning (37). Further analyses (see table 3) revealed that students' perception of achievement of the subject intended learning outcome (SILO1) was significantly correlated with the academic performance of students in the subject. Furthermore, the study confirms that students' perceived achievement of the outcome(s) may depend on what and how the subject teacher transferred subject knowledge content. The above results of the study are consistent with the findings by Ehindero and Ajibade (21) as well as Adediwura and Tayo (2). As such, hypothesis 2 is supported accordingly.

Table 4 also indicates that students' perception of teachers' pedagogical strategies was correlated positively and significantly with students' academic performance. This finding is consistent with the results of studies in the same research area: a positive relationship between teachers' pedagogical skills and students' academic performance in Social Studies was found (38) and with a significant highly positive correlation between the learning strategies and academic achievement (39). Thus, hypothesis 3 is also supported. If we look into the findings of table 4, it shows that teachers' facilitating skills were correlated positively and significantly with students' academic performance. This finding also echoes with the previous research in this direction: Centra and Potter (40) showed that teaching competences has direct linkage with students' academic results. Also, Ehindero and Ajobade (21) claimed that students' academic performance is highly relying correlated with competencies of teachers. Again, the study by Adediwura and Tayo (2) also reveals that there is a significant relationship between teachers' teaching skills and students' academic performance. Hence, hypothesis 4 is supported as expected. All in all, this study has echoed with and provided useful insight for educators and educational professions in terms of evaluation of the students' learning outcomes, pedagogical knowledge, and academic results as perceived by the students.

This study was based on the model of Four Pillars of FLIP set up in 2014 (19), which aimed to enhance students' subject knowledge and reinforce their learning experiences through interaction of educational technologies, interaction of peers, use of planned content, and facilitation of subject teachers. More specifically, the present study successfully demonstrates how the aforementioned model adopted in the flipped classroom context could influence the first-year students' perception and academic performance/outcome. What is more, it can also extend the depth of analysis of (i) participating students' responses of the subject ILO(s) before and after the intervention of flipped approach, (ii) students' perception of achievement of the subject ILO(s) and their achievement, (iii) students' perception of teachers' pedagogical knowledge and their achievement, and (iv) students' perception of teachers' facilitating skills and their achievement in the flipped classroom context. The findings show that students perceive the above factors have a positive significant relationship with their outcome performances and results.

The use of online educational technologies in teaching has been the global trend in the 21st century, and generic competencies have also been viewed essential skillsets (41). The afore-mentioned flipped earning approach provides students with opportunities to experience technology-assisted learning, in-class teamwork collaborative, and cooperative learning activities and self-study learning (42). The above flipped learning designs intend to provide practical teaching, learning, and relevant professional knowledge to learners, facilitators and/or teachers so that they can learn from the above challenges for the use of a similar pedagogical approach in their own classrooms. According to our findings, it is indicated that this FLIP model has an impact on students' subject ILOs, academic performance, and instruction. Besides, the integration of the FLIP model enables the participating students to develop collaborative learning and enhance their thinking skills (43). All in all, the flipped classroom model, (here we refer to the FLIP) with incorporation of learning and teaching designs, may be able to provide an insight for teaching professions and relevant subject teachers for further modifications, improvements, and implementations of flipped learning in different educational contexts. For example, in the recent education reform, the Ministry of Education of PRC has also highlighted the importance of inclusion of science, information technology, digital learning environments, and new instructional models (44).

As far as the limitations of the study are concerned, we have to admit that as our sample size (n = 36) is small, which may limit the generalizability of the findings. Nevertheless, it should be noted that the effect size of the significant findings is not small, hence suggesting that the findings are robust. Besides, the aim of the study is to make use of a practical FLIP model with appropriate instructional designs to enhance students' knowledge and learning experiences, and to understand how subject ILOs and pedagogies used have an impact on their academic performance. On this, we have given a strong proof to our thesis.

ACKNOWLEDGMENTS

This paper is an independent piece of manuscript based on a presentation, which, together with a conference paper titles "Integration of blended learning and flipped instruction in large classes to enhance collaborative learning between local and international students from diverse background," presented at the Asian Conference on Education in Tokyo held between 31st October and 3rd November 2018. Both endeavours are supported from the 2016 UGC Rollover Teaching Development Grant of The Hong Kong Polytechnic University, under the project title 'Addressing the University's Strategic Plan by Introducing the integration of blended learning and flipped instruction to enhance collaborative learning of large classes with diverse backgrounds between local and international students.' This chapter is a re-print of a previous publication: Chu RWC, Wong AYY, Chan MY, Shek DTL. Perceived achievement of subject learning outcomes, pedagogical strategy, facilitating skills and academic performance of university engineering students. *International Journal of Child and Adolescent Health* 2020;13(1), 23-33.

REFERENCES

[1] Allport GW. Traits revisited. Am Psychol 1966;21(1):1-10.

[2] Adediwura AA, Tayo B. Perception of teachers' knowledge, attitude and teaching skills as predictor of academic performance in Nigerian secondary school. Educ Res Rev 2007;2(7):165-71.

[3] Glover JA, Ronning RR, Bruning RH. Cognitive psychology for teachers. New York: Macmillan, 1990.

[4] James W. The principles of psychology. New York: Henry Holt, 1890.

[5] Shulman L. Knowledge and teaching: Foundations of the new reform. Harv Educ Rev 1987;57(1):1-22.

[6] Guerriero S ed. Pedagogical knowledge and the changing nature of the teaching profession. Paris: OECD Publishing, 2017. doi: https://doi.org/10.1787/9789264270695-6-en.

[7] Wilson SM, Shulman LS, Richert A. 150 different ways of knowing: Representations of knowledge in teaching. In: Calderhead J, ed. Exploring teachers' thinking. Sussex, UK: Holt Rinehart Winston, 1987:104-24.

[8] Baker JW. "The classroom flip": Using web course management tools to become the guide by the side. In 11th International Conference on College Teaching and Learning 2000;9–17.

[9] Strayer JF. How learning in an inverted classroom influences cooperation, innovation and task orientation. Learn Environ Res 2012;15:171-93. doi: https://doi: 10.1007/s10984-012-9108-4.

[10] McLuckie J, Topping KJ. Transferable skills for online peer learning. Assess Eval High Educ 2004;29(5):563-84. doi: http://dx.doi.org/10.1007/s10984-012-9108-4.

[11] Tucker B. The flipped classroom. Educ Next 2012;12(1):82. URL: https://www.educationnext.org/the-flipped-classroom/.

[12] Chen KS, Monrouxe L, Lu YH, Jenq CC, Chang YJ, Chang YC, Chai PYC. Academic outcomes of flipped classroom learning: a meta-analysis. Med Educ 2018;52:910-24. doi: https://doi: 10.1111/medu.13616.

[13] McLaughlin JE, Roth MT, Glatt DM, Gharkholonarehe N, Davidson CA, Griffin LM, Esserman DA, Mumper RJ. The flipped classroom: A course redesign to foster learning and engagement in a health professions school. Acad Med 2014;89(2):236-43.

[14] Pierce R, Fox J. Vodcasts and active-learning exercises in a "flipped classroom" model of a renal pharmacotherapy module. Am J Pharm Educ 2012;76(10):1-5, 196. doi: https://doi: 10.5688/ajpe7610196.

[15] Kavadella A, Tsiklakis K, Vougiouklakis G, Lionarakis A. Evaluation of a blended learning course for teaching oral radiology to undergraduate dental students. Eur J Dent Educ 2012;16(1):e88-95. doi: https://doi: 10.1111/j.1600-0579.2011.00680.x.

[16] Critz CM, Knight D. Using the flipped classroom in graduate nursing education. Nurse Educ 2013;38(5):210-13. doi: https://doi: 10.1097/NNE.0b013e3182a0e56a.

[17] Ruiz JG, Mintzer MJ, Leipzig RM. The impact of E-learning in medical education. Acad Med 2006;81(3):207-12.

[18] McCallin A. Interprofessional practice: learning how to collaborate. Contemp Nurse 2005;20(1):28-37.

[19] The Four Pillars of F-L-I-P™. Flipped Learning Network (FLN). URL: https://flippedlearning.org/.

[20] Farrant JS. Principles and practice of education, 2nd ed. London, UK: Longman, 2006.

[21] Ehindero OJ, Ajibade YA. What our student say about how we teach. Ife J Educ Stud 2000;7(1):1-9.

[22] Barrows HS, Tamblyn RM. Problem-based learning: an approach to medical education. New York: Springer, 1980.

[23] Barrows HS. The tutorial process. Springfield, IL: School of Medicine, Southern Illinois University, 1988.

[24] Maudsley G. Do we all mean the same thing by "problem-based learning"? A review of the concepts and a formulation of the ground rules. Acad Med 1999;74(2):178-85.

[25] Mayo WP, Donnelly MB, & Schwartz RW. Characteristics of the ideal problem-based learning tutor in clinical medicine. Eval Health Prof 1995;18:124-36.

[26] Wetzel K, Chisholm I. An evaluation of technology integration in methods courses. Technology and Teacher Education Annual. Charlottesville, VA: Association for the Advancement of Computing in Education 1996. URL: https://www.learntechlib.org/primary/p/46721/.

[27] Eggen PD, Kauchak DP. Strategies for teachers: Teaching content and thinking skills, 4th ed. Boston, MA: Allyn Bacon, 2000.

[28] Oberlander M, Jenkin N. Birth order and academic achievement. J Individ Psychol 1967;23(1):103-10.

[29] Ford DS. Self-concept and perception of school atmosphere among urban junior high school students. J Negro Educ 1985;54(1):82-8. doi: https://psycnet.apa.org/doi/10.2307/2294902.

[30] Ehigbor BO. Learners' perception of teachers' interpersonal behaviour as a predictor of academic achievement in junior secondary school certificate examination of Edo State, Nigeria. J Educ Pract 2017;8(20):144-51.

[31] Bloom BS, Engelhart MD, Furst EJ, Hill WH, Krathwohl DR. Taxonomy of educational objectives: The classification of educational goals. Handbook I: Cognitive domain. New York: David McKay, 1956.

[32] The jigsaw classroom: Jigsaw in 10 easy steps. Social Psychology Network 2019. URL: https://jigsaw.org/.

[33] Mekki TA. Cooperative learning in the EFL classroom. Special issue of the international scientific conference (2016 M-1437 e). AL-USTATH 2016:53-68.

[34] McNaught C, Leung DYP, Kember D. Report on the student engagement project. Working paper 2. Hong Kong: Centre for Learning Enhancement and Research, The Chinese University of Hong Kong, 2006. URL: https://www.researchgate.net/publication/264839865_Report_on_the_Student_Engagement_Project.

[35] Pintrich PR, Smith DAF, Duncan T, Mckeachie WJ. A manual for the use of the motivated strategies for learning questionnaire (MSLQ). ERIC IES 1991;1-79.

[36] Cartwright L, Reid M, Hammersley R, Blackburn C, Glover L. Food choice by people with intellectual disabilities at day centres: A qualitative study. J Intellect Disabil 2015;19(2):103-15. doi: https://doi: 10.1177/1744629514563423.

[37] Hew KF, Lo CK. Flipped classroom improves student learning in health professions education: A meta-analysis. BMC Med Educ 2018;18(1):1-12. URL: https://www.ncbi.nlm.nih.gov/pmc/articles/PMC5855972/pdf/12909_2018_Article_1144.pdf.

[38] Hamdan AR, Lai CL. The relationship between teachers' factors and effective teaching. Asian Soc Sci 2015;11(12):274-80. doi: http:// dx.doi:10.5539/ass.v11n12p274.

[39] Subramaniam A. Learning strategies and academic achievement among higher secondary school students. Int J Acad Res Dev 2018;3(1):864-67.

[40] Centra JA, Potteer DA. School and teacher effect: An international model. Rev Educ Res 1980;50(2):273-91. doi: http://dx.doi.org/10.3102/00346543050002273.

[41] Salpeter J. 21st century skills: Will our students be prepared? Technology and Learning-Dayton 2003;24(3):17-29.

[42] Sergis S, Zervas P, Sampson DG. ICT competence-based learning object recommendations for teachers. In the International Conference on Cognition and Exploratory Learning in Digital Age (CELDA). Porto, Portugal, 2014.

[43] Garrison DR, Anderson T, Archer W. Critical thinking, cognitive presence, and computer conferencing in distance education. Am J Distance Educ 2001;15(1):7-23.

[44] Yuan C, Moran C. Flipped classroom in China: Design, practice and implications. In HA Spires, ed. Digital transformation and innovation in Chinese education, Chap. 7. Hershey, PA: IGI Global, 2018:119-35. doi: https://doi.org/10.4018/978-1-5225-2924-8.ch007.

Appendix: Intended Learning Outcomes (ILOs) of the Subject "Light, Man and Environment" (BSE1D02)

(The following ILOs can be obtained from the subject description form (SDF) of the subject via the following link: https://www.bse.polyu.edu.hk/programmes/SubjectCode/pdf/BSE1D02.pdf)

Upon completion of the subject, students will be able to:

- ILO1 Give an account of the importance of light in their daily life;
- ILO2 Describe the nature of light and compare the properties of natural and artificial light sources;
- ILO3 Illustrate the interrelationship between light, human and the environment;
- ILO4 Explain the requirements of lighting to satisfy human biological, psychological and physiological needs; and
- ILO5 Discuss the impact of artificial lighting on people and the environment.

In: Pediatrics and Adolescent Health ISBN: 978-1-68507-490-6
Editors: J. Merrick and M. Morad

Chapter 10

GENDER OF BABY AND POSTPARTUM DEPRESSION AMONG ADOLESCENT MOTHERS IN CENTRAL JAVA, INDONESIA

Wulan Rahmadhani
and Wongsa Laohasiriwong*, PhD
Doctor of Public Health Program, Faculty of Public Health,
Khon Kaen University, Khon Kaen, Thailand
Muhammadiyah School of Health Sciences Gombong,
Central Java, Indonesia

ABSTRACT

Postpartum depression (PPD) is a major health problem of women after delivery, especially among adolescent mothers. In some cultures, the baby's gender is perceptively important, mainly among the Muslim society which is 90 percent of the population in Central Java, Indonesia. In this chapter we aimed to determine the association between gender and PPD among adolescent mothers in Central Java, Indonesia. Methods: A cross sectional study was conducted among 520 adolescent mothers who were multistage randomly selected to response to a

* Corresponding Author's E-mail: drwongsa@gmail.com.

structured questionnaire interview. The Edinburg Postpartum Depression Scale (EPDS) was administered to assess the PPD at 1-6 weeks after delivering. Multiple logistic regression was used to estimate the association between infant gender and PPD among adolescent mothers when controlling for covariates. Results: The total of 520 adolescent mothers was of an average age of 17.85±1.22 years old. The prevalence of PPD was 60.58% (95%CI: 56.29-64.70). Dissatisfaction with infant gender (Adj OR: 2.31 95%CI: 1.59-2.34), father's expected gender of the baby (Adj OR: 1.92 95%CI: 1.29-2.83), and age of the mother (Adj OR: 1.81 95%CI: 1.23-2.64) were statically significant associated with PPD. Conclusion: Postpartum depression was a common problem among adolescent mothers in Central Java, Indonesia. Furthermore, it was indicated that the gender of the baby were potential risk factors for PPD among adolescent mothers.

INTRODUCTION

Postpartum depression (PPD) is a condition where a mother who has just given birth has severe and persistent mood changes for several months or even a year or more (1). PPD is one of the most common mental disorders in Southeast Asia, particularly in Indonesia (2) with the prevalence of 50-70% (3) compared to 8-26% in United States, Japan (13.8%), Vietnam (19.4%) and 3.9% in Malaysia (4, 5). The PPD prevalence was highest among adolescent (61%) compared to adults (37.7%) mothers (6). With various changes in life, an adolescent mother is subjected to a high level of stress (7), and prone to health problems which has negative impact on their children (8).

The incidence rate of postpartum depression was 1 to 2 per 1,000 births. About 50 to 60% of women experienced postpartum depression when they had their first child, even about 50% of women who experienced postpartum had a family history of mood disorders (9). In addition, global prevalence of postpartum depression was between 10-15% (10). The rate of postpartum depression in Asia is moderately high and varies between 26-85%. For instance, in Central Java, the incidence of postpartum depression is between 50-70% (11).

PPD has multifactorial etiology including demographic and socioeconomic, medical risk factor, obstetric, psychosocial and some unique factors such as female gender of the baby and traditional rituals (1). Furthermore, the common risk factors of PPD include poverty, low social-economic status, demographic, history of pregnancy and previous history of psychiatric problems, poor relationship with the mother-in-law, giving birth with female gender and dissatisfaction with baby's gender (12). However, the role of baby's gender satisfaction is different across the cultures (13). A study in Western countries reported that there was no association between baby's gender satisfactions and PPD (14), yet different findings which were discovered among studies in India (15), Iran (16) and Nigeria (17) indicated that there was a significant association between gender of baby satisfaction and PPD. But little is known about factor predictor postpartum depression in adolescent mothers.

OUR STUDY

A cross-sectional was conducted among postpartum adolescent mothers in Central Java, Indonesia. The sample size of 520 was calculated based on the formula of Hsieh et al. (18). A multi-stage random sampling was administered to select the samples. First, three districts were randomly selected and secondly, six sub districts were selected from the three districts. In addition, 520 adolescent mothers were randomly selected from each sub district proportional to size of the population. The inclusion criteria were a mother who delivered a baby before the age of 20 years, had delivered a baby within six weeks, and had good verbal communication with the researcher, were literate with a good read and write ability and willing to participate in this study. The exclusion criteria was those who were severely ill physiologically and mentally, mothers with illicit drug use and past history of severe mental disorders.

Before beginning data collection, the researcher distributed document to participants for the informed consent. Adolescent mothers who submitted participant consent with the signature were included in the study.

The research tool was a structured questionnaire developed from the literature reviews relevant to the research questions. The question consisted of three parts including: 1) demographic and socioeconomic characteristics: age, marital status, education attainment, occupational, types of area staying, type of household, family size, family monthly income, average expenditure monthly, and financial situation; 2) latest pregnancy conditions: planned pregnancy, wanted pregnancy, awareness of pregnancy, gestational age at first ANC (antenatal care) visit, times of ANC visits, type of delivery, gender of baby, mother's expectation of baby, spouse's expected gender of baby and satisfied with gender of baby 3) PPD was screened by using the Edinburg Postnatal Depression Scale (EPDS) questionnaire. The EPDS was a ten-item self-administered questionnaire which consisted of 10 questions. Questions number 1,2 and 4 was with sign (*) with Likert scale of 0,1,2,3, whereas questions number 3,5,6,7,8,9 and 10 with Likert scale 3,2,1,0. The maximal score of the EPDS were 30 and interpreted as a dichotomous outcome with cutoff point of ≥13 as has PPD and <13 as 'does not have PPD' (1). The questionnaires were tested by three experts for content validity. The reliability test was conducted among 30 adolescent mothers in Gombong, Kebumen Central Java, the Cronbach's alpha coefficient of the EPDS was 0.89.

All data were transferred to an excel file and then moved to STATA (Version 13.1) software for data analysis. Demographic, socioeconomic characteristics and latest pregnancy conditions of the respondents were described presenting frequency and percentage for categorical data, and mean, standard deviation, or median, minimum and maximum for continuous data. Simple logistic regression was used for bivariate analysis to explore the association between each individual factor and PDD presenting crude odds (OR) and 95% confident interval (95%CI). The variable that the bivariate analysis has p-value <0.25 was then included in the multivariable analysis. Multiple logistic regression were carried out to estimate the association of multiple variables and PPD presenting adjusted odds ratio (Adj. OR) and 95%CI at statistical significance levels of 0.05.

Table 1. Demographic and socioeconomics characteristics of Adolescent mother in Central Java, Indonesia

Demographic and socioeconomics characteristics	Number	Percentage
Age		
<17	92	17.69
17-18	188	36.15
19	240	46.15
Mean ± SD = 17.85±1.22; Median (Min-Max) = 18 (15-19)		
Marital status		
Married with marriage certificate	217	41.73
Married without marriage certificate	303	58.27
Education attainment		
No formal education	1	0.19
Primary School	24	4.62
Secondary school	413	79.42
High school	82	15.77
Occupational		
Housewife	390	75.00
Unskilled worker	130	25.00
Type of area of staying		
Urban	318	61.15
Rural	202	38.85
Types of household		
Extended family	383	73.65
Nuclear family	124	23.85
Living alone	13	2.50
Family size (Persons)		
<4	137	26.35
4-6	218	41.92
>7	165	31.73
Mean ± SD	5.76±2.18	
Median (Min-Max)	6 (3-13)	
Family average monthly income (in USD)		
37 -73	300	57.69
74- 148	160	30.77
>149	60	11.54
Mean ± SD	98.7 ± 42.8	
Median (Min-Max)	74.1(37-185.2)	
Average expenditure monthly (in USD)		
37 73	307	59.04
74- 148	154	29.62
>149	59	11.54
Mean ± SD	98.7 ± 42.8	
Median (Min-Max)	74.1(37-185.2)	
Financial situation		
Enough without saving	433	83.27
Enough with saving	51	9.81
Not Enough	24	4.62
Not enough with debts	12	2.31

Clinical Ethical permission for the study was obtained from the Committee on Research the office of Khon Kaen University Ethics Committee in human research with number HE602348.

Table 2. Latest pregnancy conditions of adolescent mothers in Central Java, Indonesia

Latest pregnancy conditions	Number	Percentage
Planned Pregnancy		
Yes	316	60.77
No	204	39.23
Wanted Pregnancy		
Yes	316	60.77
No	204	39.23
Awareness of pregnancy		
No menstruation	371	71.35
Pregnancy test	75	14.42
Nausea vomiting	74	14.23
Gestational age of first ANC visit		
<12	137	26.35
≥12	383	73.65
Mean ± SD	17.74 ± 7.34	
Median (Min-Max)	20 (4-28)	
Number of ANC visits		
<4	326	62.69
≥4	194	37.31
Mean ± SD	6.59 ± 5.70	
Median (Min-Max)	3 (2-16)	
Type of Delivery		
Normal	414	79.62
Caesarea	106	20.38
Gender of Baby		
Female	261	50.19
Male	259	49.81
Mother expected baby gender		
Male	261	50.19
Female	259	49.81
Father expected baby gender		
Male	325	62.50
Female	195	37.50
Satisfaction with baby gender		
No	316	60.77
Yes	204	39.23

FINDINGS

A total of 520 adolescent mothers aged 17.85 ±1.22 years old participated in the study. The majority were without marriage certificate (58.27%). Most of the respondents finished secondary school (42%), with their occupation as housewife (75.00%). 61.15% lived in urban areas and 73.65% had extended family (73.65%) with an average of family size of 5.76±2.18 persons. Their average monthly family income was 74.1(37-185.2) US$ with an average monthly expenditure of 98.7 ± 42.8 US$. Most of the adolescent mothers had enough income without any saving (83.27%). All of the respondents were Muslim.

Latest pregnancy conditions

Most of the adolescent mothers had both planned pregnancy and wanted pregnancy (60.77%), respectively. Missed period were the most common sign for the pregnant women to perceive being pregnant (71.35%), followed by pregnancy test (14.42%) and nausea vomiting (14.23%). Only 26.35% had the first ANC before 12 weeks and 37.31% had at least four ANC visits. Most of the mothers had normal delivery (79.62%). The gender of the delivered babies were male gender for 50.19%. 62.50% of the fathers expected to have a male baby whereas only 50.19% of the mothers expected a male baby gender (50.19%). 60.77% of the adolescent mothers were dissatisfied with the gender of the baby.

Postpartum depression situation

Based on the Edinburg Postnatal Depression Scale (EPDS) 60.58% (95%CI: 56.29-64.70) of the adolescent mothers had PPD.

Table 3. Prevalence of postpartum depression among adolescent mothers in Central Java, Indonesia

Postpartum depression	**Number**	**Percentage**	**95% CI**
Postpartum depression			
Depression (≥13 scores)	315	60.58	56.29-64.70
No depression (<13 scores)	205	39.42	27.70-35.29
Mean ± SD	12.80±7.52		
Median (Min-Max)	13(2-22)		

The simple logistic regression indicated factors that were possibly associated with PPD among adolescent mothers with p-value <0.25 were: age, types of household, family size, average monthly family income, gestation age at first ANC visit, father expected baby's gender, mother expected baby gender, satisfaction with baby's gender. These factors were then preceded to the multivariable analysis (see Table 4).

Multivariable analysis of factors associated with postpartum depression among adolescent mother: A multiple logistic regression

The final model of multivariable analysis using a multiple logistic regression indicated that the adolescent mothers that were dissatisfied with gender of baby had 2.31 times higher odds of having PDD when compared to those who were satisfied with the gender of the baby (Adj.OR = 2.31; 95%CI: 1.59-2.34; p-value: <0.001). Other factors which also had influence on PDD among adolescent mothers were spouse's expected a female baby's gender (Adj. OR = 1.92; 95%CI: 1.29-2.83; p-value < 0.001), they were younger than 18 years old for the latest pregnancy (Adj. OR = 1.81; 95%CI: 1.23-2.64; p-value < 0.002) (see Table 5).

Table 4. Bivariate analysis of factors associated with postpartum depression among adolescent mother: a simple logistic regression

Factors	Number	% of PPD	Crude OR	95%CI	p-value
Overall	**520**	**60.58**	**N/A**	**56.29-64.70**	**N/A**
Age					
<18	310	55.48	1		0.004
>18	210	68.10	1.71	1.18-2.47	
Types of Household					
Nuclear family	137	13.87	1		<0.001
Extended family	383	77.28	12.31	12.31-36.28	
Family size (person)					
≥7	283	75.23	1		<0.001
<6	237	43.04	4.02	2.77-5.84	
Family average monthly income					
< 111 USD	300	55.67	1		0.008
≥ 111 USD	220	67.27	1.63	1.13-2.35	
Gestation age at first ANC visit					
<12	137	23.36	1		<0.001
≥ 12	383	73.89	9.28	5.88-14.66	
Mother's expectation on gender on the baby					
Female	259	54.44	1		0.004
Male	261	66.67	1.67	1.17-2.38	
Spouse's expectation on gender on the baby					
Male	325	55.38	1		
Female	195	69.23	1.81	1.24-2.63	0.002
Satisfaction with baby gender					
Yes	316	48.04	1		<0.001
No	204	68.67	2.37	1.64-3.40	

* Simple logistic regression (SLR) shows crude OR ** Multilevel logistic regression shows Adjusted OR:95%CI and p-value after adjusted for other covariates factors.

Table 5. Multivariable analysis of factors associated with postpartum depression among adolescent mother: a multiple logistic regression

Variables	Total Number		*SLR	**Multilevel logistic regression		
		%	OR	OR	95%CI	p-value
		PPD	Crude	Adjust		
Satisfaction with baby gender						
Yes	204	48.04	1			<0.001
No	316	68.67	2.37	2.31	1.23-2.64	
Spouse expectation on gender of a baby						
Male	325	55.38	1			0.001
Female	195	69.23	1.81	1.92	1.29-2.83	
Age of the mothers						
≥18	210	55.48	1			0.002
<18	310	68.10	1.71	1.81	1.23-3.34	

Discussion

The prevalence of postpartum depression among the adolescent mother in Central Java, Indonesia was 60.58%. This PPD was identified by a screening tool for PDD. The Edinburgh Postnatal Depression Scale (EPDS) was developed to assist health professionals in detecting mothers suffering from PPD, which is a distressing disorder. It is indicated that it is more prolonged than the "blues" that can occur in the first week after delivery. There is a need to further confirm diagnosis, however, most importantly prompt and appropriate interventions are able to solve their PPD problem. The possible explanation was that these mothers were not yet mature since they were younger than 20 years old at delivery a baby. This was confirmed by the multivariable analysis which will be discussed further.

In this study, it was investigated the relationship between gender of baby satisfaction and PPD among adolescent mothers. Gender of baby is an important issue and one of the major problems in some cultures (19). Studies indicated its influences on antepartum and postpartum depression in many countries (18). Modification of health behaviors to prevent postpartum depression is an obligation to a better health of adolescent mothers. Ahmed et al. (20) mentioned that disappointment of mothers can be caused by rejection from the mothers of her baby. However, many of the mothers expressed rarely her hopelessness to their spouses, families and close friends. The current study found that baby gender dissatisfaction was significantly associated with PDD (Adj. OR: 2.31; 95% CI: 1.59-2.34; p-value: <0.001). About half had a female baby (50.19%). Many adolescent mothers were disappointed with the gender of their baby, because the baby's gender did not match with adolescent mother's expectations, which was also found in the study by Alizadeh et al. (21). They found that there was a significant association between neonatal gender and postpartum depression with p-value 0.002. A study by Tychey et al. (22) also indicated the gender of baby as an influencing factors of postpartum depression with p-value = 0.04. Being unhappy with the gender of the baby was a significant factors in postpartum depression (23). It was asserted that some studies reported PPD higher if the gender of baby were females among the patriarchal family type (24). For instance, in Central Java, Indonesia, most of the families were patriarchal type. Therefore, male gender is more preferable. Our study found that most of the spouses expected a male baby (62.50%). spouse's expected of female baby increased the odds of PPD (Adj. OR = 1.92; 95%CI: 1.29-2.83; p-value: 0.001). The expectation of the gender of the baby became one of the major risk factors for postpartum depression.

Furthermore, it was also found that the younger adolescent mothers (aged <18 years old) had higher odds of having PPD (Adj. OR = 1.81; 95%CI: 1.23-2.64; p-value: 0.002). In the term of psychological readiness, young adolescents are too young for motherhood and caring for the baby (25). Crisis situations, unready to be a parent and the social environment are problems among women who gave birth at a young age (26). Some adolescent mothers found that the period after delivery of their babies as a difficult period causing emotional stress. El-Hachem (27) suggested age as a factor for predisposing PPD, especially the delivery of a baby under the age of 20 years old.

CONCLUSION

Most of the adolescent mothers in Central Java have suffered from PPD. There is actually an association between dissatisfaction of the baby's gender and PPD among adolescent mothers. Other influencing factors of PPD were age of mothers and spouse's expectation of baby's gender.

Intervention research on how to prevent PPD in the community is essential. Social interactions and counseling during antenatal and postpartum cares are important to prevent and solve PPD. Health care professional should help to provide proactive and holistic care which can focus on not only physical but also psychological and social function for the couple, family and community.

Limitation and strength of study

A cross sectional study could only identify the factors associated with PPD, cross sectional study also could not predict the cause and effect in depression. Another limitation was the EPDS, which is a screening questionnaire and not a diagnostic instrument. Therefore further actions are needed. The questionnaires did not mention previous history of depression, mental illness and family history about depression. Therefore, it might be considered being predictive symptom of depression. The strength of this study was that the samples were a regional representative which could be generalized to the population in Central Java. This study used a standardized instrument which had high reliabilities in our setting of 0.89 to screening depression (EPDS).

ACKNOWLEDGEMENTS

We acknowledge all the adolescent mothers whose cooperation and understanding made the study possible. This research was financially supported by the Research and Training Center for Enhancing Quality of Life for Working-Age People, Khon Kaen University, Thailand.

REFERENCES

[1] Shivalli S, Gururaj N. Postnatal depression among rural women in south India: Do socio-demographic, obstetric and pregnancy outcome have a role to play? PLoS One 2015;10(4):e0122079.

[2] Heh SS. Postpartum depression. J Nurs 2013;41:30-36.

[3] Muslihatun WN. Asuhan neonatus bayi dan balita. Yogyakarta: Fitramaya, 2014.

[4] Miyake Y, Tanaka K, Sasaki S, Hirota Y. Employment, income, and education and risk of postpartum depression: The Osaka maternal and child health study. J Affec Disord 2011;130:133-7.

[5] O'Hara MW, Swain AM. Rates and risk of postpartum depression: A meta-analysis. Inter Rev Psychiatry 1996;8:37-54.

[6] Wang SY, Jiang XY, Jan WC, Chen CH. A comparative study of postnatal depression and its predictors in Taiwan and mainland China. Am J Obstet Gynecol 2003;189:1407-12.

[7] Lara MA, Berenzon S, García FJ, Medina-Mora ME, Rey GN, Ameth J, et al. Population study of depressive symptoms and risk factors in pregnant and parenting Mexican adolescents. Rev Panam Salud Publica 2012;31:102-8.

[8] Liang ELM. Adolescent pregnancy: A review of the evidence. New York: UNFPA, 2013.

[9] Keshavarzi F, Yazdchi K, Rahimi M, Rezaei M, Farnia V, Davarinejad O, et al. Post partum depression and thyroid function. Iran J Psychiatry 2011;6:117-20.

[10] Motzfeldt I, Andreasen S, Pedersen AL, Pedersen ML. Prevalence of postpartum depression in Nuuk, Greenland - A cross-sectional study using edinburgh postnatal depression scale. Int J Circumpolar Health 2013;72:10.3402/ ijch.v72i0.21114.

[11] Manuaba I. Memahami Kesehatan Reproduksi Wanita. Jakarta: Arcan, 2010.

[12] Gausia K, Ryder D, Ali M, Fisher C, Moran A, Koblinsky M. Obstetric complications and psychological well-being: Experiences of Bangladeshi women during pregnancy and childbirth. J Health Popul Nutr 2012;30:172-80.

[13] Goldbort J. Transcultural analysis of postpartum depression. MCN Am J Maternal Child Nurs 2006;31:121-6.

[14] Stewart DE, Robertson E, Dennis C-L, Grace SL, Tamara W. Postpartum depression: Literature review of risk factors and interventions. Toronto: Toronto Public Health 2003:9-70.

[15] Patel V, Andrade C. Pharmacological treatment of severe psychiatric disorders in the developing world: Lessons from India. CNS Drugs 2003;17:1071-80.

[16] Kheirabadi GR, Maracy MR, Barekatain M, Salehi M, Sadri GH, Kelishadi M, et al. Risk factors of postpartum depression in rural areas of Isfahan province, Iran. Arch Iran Med 2009;12:461-7.

[17] Abiodun OA. Postnatal depression in primary care populations in Nigeria. Gen Hosp Psychiatry 2006;28:133-6.

[18] Rodgers A, Atuhairwe S. M129 revitalization of ppiud insertion in Uganda: Integrating delivery and family planning services. Inte J Gynecol Obstet 2012;119:S161-S900.

[19] Senturk V, Abas M, Berksun O, Stewart R. Social support and antenatal depression in extended and nuclear family environments in Turkey: A cross-sectional survey. BMC Psychiatry 2011;24:11-48.

[20] Ahmed HM, Alalaf SK, Al-Tawil NG. Screening for postpartum depression using Kurdish version of edinburgh postnatal depression scale. Arch Gynecol Obstet 2012;285:1249-55.

[21] Shamshiri Milani H, Azargashb E, Beyraghi N, Defaie S, Asbaghi T. Effect of telephone-based support on postpartum depression: A randomized controlled trial. Int J Fertil Steril 2015;9:247-253.

[22] De Tychey C, Briançon S, Lighezzolo J, Spitz E, Kabuth B, De Luigi V, et al. Quality of life, postnatal depression and baby gender. J Clin Nurs 2008;17:312-22.

[23] Cooper PJ, Tomlinson M, Swartz L, Woolgar M, Murray L, Molteno C. Post-partum depression and the mother-infant relationship in a South African peri-urban settlement. Br J Psychiatry 1999;175:554-8.

[24] Xie RH, He G, Koszycki D, Walker M, Wen SW. Fetal sex, social support, and postpartum depression. Can J Psychiatry 2009;54:750-6.

[25] Khodaverdi F, Alhani F, Kazemnejad A, Khodaverdi Z. The relationship between obesity and quality of life in school children. Front Psychol 2011;31:39-44.

[26] Gaillard A, Le Strat Y, Mandelbrot L, Keïta H, Dubertret C. Predictors of postpartum depression: Prospective study of 264 women followed during pregnancy and postpartum. Psychiatr Res 2014;215:341-6.

[27] El-Hachem C, Rohayem J, Bou Khalil R, Richa S, Kesrouani A, Gemayel R, et al. Early identification of women at risk of postpartum depression using the Edinburgh Postnatal Depression Scale (EPDS) in a sample of Lebanese women. BMC Psychiatry 2014;14:242.

In: Pediatrics and Adolescent Health ISBN: 978-1-68507-490-6
Editors: J. Merrick and M. Morad

Chapter 11

THE ASSOCIATION BETWEEN SELF-REGULATION AND VIOLENT PROPENSITIES AMONG SAUDI GIRLS

Uhuud Alassaf*

Department of Human Development and Psychoeducational Studies,
School of Education, Howard University,
Washington DC, USA

ABSTRACT

There is limited research on Saudi girls' self-regulation and violent propensities and attitudes in Saudi Arabia. Recent statistics on bullying in Saudi schools noted a noticeable increase warranting the attention of not only educators, but also the mental health community to propose culturally sensitive compatible interventions capable of redressing deficiencies in self-regulation and violent tendencies in schools. This research investigates the association between improved self-regulation and decreased violent behaviors among adolescents in a new cultural context, Saudi school girls (11-15 years). Further, it investigates

* Corresponding Author's E-mail: Afs_assaf@hotmail.com.

whether income levels moderate such an association. Using a sample of 132 girls from Jeddah and correlational methods, the association between self-regulation and an index of attitudes against violence was moderate, $r = 0.42$. Findings of this research suggests that Saudi girls possess low levels of self-regulation and moderate to high levels of violent tendencies requiring immediate attention. The paper highlights the importance of counseling services and therapy in addressing such deficiencies. More importantly, the discussion section reviews recent evaluations and assessments of new therapies including creative, art, music and mindfulness treatments and their positive significant effects in increasing self-regulation and decreasing violent behaviors among adolescents. This analysis paves the road for further empirical study of adolescent attitudes and behaviors in Saudi Arabia, a still emerging field in psychology and education.

INTRODUCTION

Attitudes and behaviors related to violence, aggressiveness, and bullying carry both short and long-term negative consequences for the physical, mental, social, and academic growth of adolescents. Peers in school pressure each other through a variety of ways, including verbal bullying, physical infliction of harm, victimization, and discrimination. Victims of school-related aggressive behaviors such as these have been shown to develop increased insecurities and anxiety in comparison to other students (1). Being subjected to violent or aggressive acts in schools has also been associated with a wide range of internalizing problems (2). Victims of school aggression also seem to be less equipped for adapting to new environments and therefore suffer from heightened emotional distress that disenables them from feeling empathy toward others in future social interactions (3). The phenomenon of increasing aggressive behavior has necessitated immediate governmental interventions globally, including in the developing world. Nevertheless, research has been limited regarding the antecedents and consequences of school violence, in all its forms, on victims in quickly developing nations. Violence in schools has only recently received attention and interventions in fast-paced developing nations like the Kingdom of Saudi Arabia. A recent survey of adolescent health needs in the Kingdom of Saudi Arabia concluded that about 25% of school children have been exposed to some form of bullying during the thirty days prior to the commissioning of the study. While boys have been shown to bully each other more than girls, the difference was not very high (27% versus 22%), raising concerns about the safety of not only boys' schools but also those of girls which have often been thought to be much safer in comparison to the educational institutions of the opposite gender (4). In a retrospective questionnaire investigating the prevalence of violence in Saudi schools, adults reported high rates of exposure (ranging from 28% for males and 15% for females) (5). Note that such figures are likely to be misrepresentative since such actions are prone to being under-reported by respondents due to a plethora of reasons such as stigma. Given this frequency, researchers and educators have sought to utilize behavioral interventions to curb the development and maintenance of violence-prone attitudes and behaviors in schools.

Self-regulation constitutes one of the most widely cited remedies for controlling and preventing school violence in its various forms (6). If students are actively engaged in methods of self-control instead of fighting, bullying, victimizing, discriminating, and engaging in other forms of violence among themselves, the phenomenon is likely to be mitigated. To do so, their self-efficacy, motivation, desire, and skills for addressing violence in school settings must be developed. Prior research has also shown that a robustly positive statistical correlation exists between self-regulation and empathy, amicability, and non-aggressive forms of conflict resolution among adolescents (7).

National samples from the United States, Canada, Spain, Italy, and Israel have further demonstrated that higher emotional self-control is associated with less aggressive tendencies and actions in schools (8). Investigation of the association between self-regulation and aggression among adolescents in the developing world is still in its infancy, however. This study explores, therefore, the relationships between adolescent girls in Saudi schools by utilizing an original dataset collected in 2018 from public and private schools across the country. The present study finds a robust association between self-regulation and aggressive attitudes among Saudi girls. Higher levels of self-regulation, across all its dimensions: cognitive, emotional and behavioral, are associated with lower levels of aggression. This relationship is not affected by income levels, and is likely to exist regardless of demographic characteristics. Further, results indicate that Saudi girls possess low levels of self-regulation and moderate to high levels of aggressive attitudes. Such psychological needs require immediate interventions from educators, the government, and parents. A host of well-established therapies, such as cognitive based therapies and new, innovative, therapeutic treatments that include creativity, art, music, and mindfulness interventions are available to address the needs of Saudi girls. This analysis sheds light on the mental health needs of adolescent Saudi females, a group that is often seldom researched or considered in empirical psychological analyses in Saudi Arabia.

LITERATURE REVIEW

Self-regulation improves adolescents' educational performance, emotional well-being, social bonding, and economic fortunes (2). This refers to the management and control of one's feelings, observations, and actions in order to facilitate conducive behaviors directed by clear and well-defined goals. Higher levels of self-regulation have been associated with lower likelihoods of engaging in deviant behaviors such as drug abuse, aggression, bullying, alcoholism, and suicide. Recent neuroscientific evidence has suggested that the period of adolescence (11-15 years of age) witnesses extensive shifts in brain development, reflecting the need for investment in self-regulation at this stage. Systems of reward and emotional exploration evolve much faster in comparison to the physical brain architecture tasked with higher order organization and planning. Therefore, interventions aiming to increase self-regulation levels should target adolescents, particularly among vulnerable groups which suffer from exposure to risk factors for psychopathologies (9).

Self-regulation is not static and changes throughout one's lifespan. It is acquired by instruction, social learning, and the interaction of personal, environmental, and social contexts. Researchers have dissected the meta concept into three distinct types: emotional, cognitive, and behavioral. Each distinct set of knowledge, skills, and abilities can be transmitted through formal learning institutions, at home through caregivers, and socially through the adoption of favorable attitudes and practices (10). One of the main antecedents to the construction of healthy levels of self-regulation is the presence of a supportive environment. The buttressing effect of institutions, family, peers, and the predictability and responsiveness of the environment enables adolescents to better acquire self-regulation (11).

Bandura (12) proposed the social cognitive theory, suggesting that individuals learn through the observation of others and the consequences of their actions. This contrasted with earlier psychological theories by assuming that appropriate learning could only be accomplished through direct experience. Bandura observed that individuals utilize their environments, behaviors, and emotions in learning new skills or abilities. The process of learning goes, therefore, through four stages according to Bandura: attention, retention, reproduction, and motivation. Throughout the learning process Bandura suggested that self-regulation (the ability to self-generate ideas, perceptions, plans, and feelings that manage the learning process in hopes of achieving the intended goals) is set by the learner.

Self-regulation and aggression

Prior research on self-regulation and aggressive behavior has established a robustly positive correlation between low levels of self-control, emotional regulation, and overall self-regulation with incidences of aggressive attitudes and behaviors. In their seminal work resulting from five experiments, DeWall et al. (13) tested the effect of depletion in self-regulation on aggression. The five experiments conducted by the authors utilized various settings, including different measurements of aggression and different depletion tools for self-regulation in each experiment. Main findings of these studies were that people whose self-regulation depleted showed more aggression than those who did not experience the decrease, especially in the face of provocation. In the first experiment, participants were randomly assigned to the experimental and control groups before being told that they were in a taste-preference study. In the experimental group, participants were asked to sit in front of a donut without eating it for a specified time while the control group was placed in front of a less appealing food choice (a radish). Participants were then asked to write an essay on their food preferences. All participants were told that they were paired with a partner of the same sex in the next room, and their essays would be evaluated by the partner. After participants finished the essays, the experimenter came in with a very negative evaluation of the participant's work (which the participant believed came from their anonymous partner) stating that "this is one of the worst essays I've ever read." Upon this provocation, the participants were asked to prepare a snack for the partner who gave the negative evaluation of the essay. Each participant was provided with chips, an empty bowl, and hot sauce with a label stating spicy. In the partner's taste preferences list, spicy was selected as the least favorite food. Knowing this, the participant prepared the snack by putting a certain amount of spice of their choice on the cracker. The authors found that those who were depleted in self-regulation by sitting in front of a donut for hours put more spice on the cracker than those who were not depleted in self-regulation. This experiment showed that ego-depletion leads to aggressive behavior.

The authors examined the rival hypothesis by testing the strength of provocation or insult on the incidence of aggressive behavior (13). To accomplish this, the authors added a no-insult control condition in the second and third experiments with the participant receiving praise instead of criticism for their essays. Different manipulations were also used for self-regulation depletion, such as having the participants control their attention from distractions while watching a video and overriding their natural tendency to read a word printed in a different color than its semantic meaning (i.e., the word red printed in the color green). The authors also used different measures for aggression, such as sending a disruptive and noisy voice through a computer game and thwarting the partner's opportunity for gaining a scholarship by writing a negative candidate evaluation. Both experiments confirmed that depletion in self-regulation along with a provocation lead to increased aggression. In their fourth experiment, the authors aimed to strengthen their conclusion while assessing the participants' tendency for aggressive behaviors by using a hypothetical real-life situation instead of a laboratory setting. Results of the experiment confirmed the first three studies, asserting that depleted participants showed greater levels of aggression in the face of a provocation. In this experiment, the authors also controlled for one additional variable: trait self-control. Findings revealed that the interaction between trait self-control and depletion condition explained the participants' intention to aggress. The results further showed that depleted participants who were low in self-control exhibited a greater level of aggression ($b = 44.81$, $p = .01$), while participants who were high in trait self-control did not present a significant level of aggression ($b = -16.75$, $p = .37$). Trait self-control was measured by the brief version of the scale posited by Tangney et al. (14).

In the last experiment, the participants were asked to write about one successful aggressive restraint in which they were able to withhold their urge to aggress and then another on an unsuccessful attempt to restrain aggressiveness. Upon completing these essays, the participants were asked to fill out a modified version of the State Depletion Scale in order to measure their level of depletion at the time of the event (15). The results revealed that a significant amount of the aggressive behaviors reported by participants were preceded by self-regulation depletion, $t(136) = 2.73$, $p = .007$. More importantly, the fourth and fifth experiments revealed that depletion of self-regulation itself, without insulting or provocation, does not have a significant effect on aggression. Accordingly, participants receiving praise for their essays did not show significant aggression although their self-regulation had been depleted. The second experiment yielded results of $F(1, 51) = 2.91$, $p < .11$ for those who had received praise for their essays. The third experiment, by the same token, did not find significant levels of aggression among depleted participants when there was no provocation.

Summarizing the experimental evidence on the relationship between self-regulation and aggression, Inzlicht and Schmeichel (16) attempted to provide a conceptual model for the established hypothesis in the literature that depletion of self-control at Time 1 leads to a reduction in performance of self-control at Time 2. According to the authors (16), this notion explains the relationship between ego depletion and aggression and has been confirmed by many studies in the extant literature across a variety of experimental settings (e.g., 13). However, Inzlicht and Schmeichel also argue that what is missing in the literature is the mechanism of ego depletion. According to their conceptual model, self-control depletion at Time 2 is simply due to shifts in motivation, attention, and emotion. In this regard the authors criticize the existing experiments (despite being from multiple perspectives) since they ignore the shift in motivation and attention. This first criticism comes as a result of most experiments offering little or no incentive for the participants' performance at Time 1. Because of this, they do not receive enough benefit for self-controlling at Time 1. As a result, this decreases their motivation to control themselves further at the next phase. Therefore, the authors call the readers' attention to the need for controlling the mediation effect of low motivation on regulation in future studies. The authors go on to suggest the increased strength to act with impulse as an alternative meditative factor resulting in aggression that is not included in other studies. Their belief is that depletion in self-regulation may increase the motivation for impulsive actions (following of urges and desires). The third factor the authors state is not accounted for in other studies is that ego depletion may be due more to shifts in participants' attention of when to regulate rather than their inability to exert control. The logic behind this idea is that people may fail to grasp when regulation and control are required due to their shifted attention during experiments. Overall, the authors claim that self-control depletion occurs due to shifts in motivation and attention, and they call fellow researchers to consider their conceptual model in order to provide new studies with more explanatory power.

Non-experimental longitudinal and cross-sectional studies from around the world have also confirmed the negative correlation between self-regulation and aggressive attitudes and behaviors among adolescents. Castillo et al. (17) studied the effect of emotional intelligence interventions on the level of aggression and empathy among adolescents in Spain. They conducted a quasi-experiment with a pre-test post-test model utilizing a total of 590 adolescents consisting of middle and high school students (aged between 11 and 17) over the period of two academic years (2009 and 2010). Three hundred and sixty-one of the participants were randomly assigned to the experimental group, while 229 were assigned to a control group. The experimental group was exposed to the emotional intelligence intervention known as the INTEMO program, which is an academic curriculum aiming to increase students' skills in perceiving, facilitating, understanding, and regulating emotions. Meanwhile, the control group was not exposed to any such interventions. The authors measured aggression and empathy with self-reporting questionnaires: the Spanish version of the Aggression Questionnaire and the Interpersonal Reactivity Index (18, 19). Aggression was measured by multiple variables, including physical aggression, verbal aggression, hostility, and anger. Empathy, on the other hand, was measured by fantasy, perspective taking, empathic concern, and personal distress. The findings of the study revealed that those who participated in the intervention reported less aggression and more empathy in most scales, while those in the control group did not show a significant difference in their aggressive and empathetic behaviors. Although Castillo et al. showed a significant decrease in aggression after the emotional intelligence intervention generally, the findings did not lend much support to the physical and verbal aggression scales.

Similarly, Franken et al. (6) concluded that adolescents with low self-control develop externalizing behaviors, including violent attitudes, at a faster rate in comparison to those who have higher levels of self-regulation. Using the Social Network Analysis of Risk behavior in Early adolescents (SNARE), the authors found support for their hypothesis that a negative association exists between self-regulation, cognitive, behavioral, emotional, and a wide range of externalizing behaviors (including aggressive perceptions and actions). Franken et al. stated, "To test our hypotheses, the role of self-control was estimated in the behavior dynamics....Testing our first hypothesis, in two of the four networks self-control was negatively associated with the development of externalizing behavior [negative effect form self-control, School 1 Cohort 2 *b* (*SE*) = -0.61 (0.20), School 2 Cohort 1 *b*(*SE*) = -0.47 (0.23)]" (6). The authors continued to argue that the effect of externalizing behaviors by an adolescents' friends do not have a significant effect on the low self-control and high externalizing behaviors group, contradicting many of the earlier studies that cited a positive connection between peers' violent behaviors and an adolescents' development of new violent attitudes. Therefore, interventions should focus more on the adolescents beginning with low self-control.

Özdemir, Vazsonyi and Cok (20) also tested both the direct and indirect relationship between parenting processes, low self-control, and aggression. They conducted a survey among 546 adolescents, aged 14-18 years, attending high schools in Turkey. In the survey, parenting processes are measured by the Adolescent Family Process which consists of 30 items for maternal and 30 items for paternal factors across six distinct dimensions (closeness, support, monitoring, communication, conflict, and peer approval). Self-control is measured by a scale with 24 items put forward by Grasmick, Tittle, Bursik and Arneklev. Aggression is then measured by the aggression questionnaires proposed by Buss and Perry (18). Results of the study revealed that all parental and maternal processes were negatively associated with both low self-control and aggression. Moreover, low self-control was positively and significantly associated with aggression (r = .45). After running a structural equation model, the authors found that there was no direct effect by parental and maternal processes on aggression, but they had an indirect effect on aggression through low self-control.

The association between self-regulation and aggressive attitudes and behaviors is consistent across varying adolescent groups, regardless of gender, race, ethnicity, or nationality. Watson et al. (22) assessed the merit of two explanations for the development of violent attitudes and behaviors among adolescents. They found support for two pathways to violence: the severe risk-factors effect and the cumulative effect. The first, consisted of a host of risk characteristics (including incohesive families, authoritarian parenting, low levels of regulatory control, and chronic stress). In the second pathway, aggressive behavior is manifested later in adolescence due to the accumulative effect of all risk factors. The authors did not specifically focus on the role of self-regulation as a main factor. However, they highlighted its potential effect as a main variable in driving violent attitudes and behaviors among adolescents.

McLaughlin et al. (9) longitudinally investigated the relationship between emotional dysregulation and psychopathology among a large sampling of adolescents (N = 1,065). They found support for the claim that increased emotional dysregulation is associated with the development and sustenance of aggressive attitudes and behaviors among adolescents. Their structural equation model results indicated that "Time 1 emotion dysregulation was significantly associated with Time 2 symptoms of anxiety ($\beta = .19, p < .001$), aggression ($\beta = .18, p < .001$), and eating pathology ($\beta = .20, p < .001$), controlling for Time 1 symptomatology" (9). This result confirms earlier cross-sectional findings exhibiting a robustly negative association between self-regulation and both aggressive expression and conduct among children and adults.

In the same fashion, Cuccì et al. (23) tested the mediating effect of emotional dysregulation on the relationship between exposure to authoritarian parenting styles and violent dating behavior among adolescents. They modelled the relationship separately for males and females. Using self-reported data from 622 Italian adolescents, the authors found support for their expected claim, namely a positive mediating effect existing between emotional dysregulation and violence in dating caused by memories from authoritarian parenting styles experienced during early childhood. Heleniak, et al. (11) analyzed the mediating effect of emotional dysregulation on the development of internalizing negative behavioral symptoms, including violent attitudes. They desired to substantiate the claim that emotional dysregulation mediates the relationship between exposure to community violence and the exhibition of violent perceptions and actions individually. Using a diverse sample of 267 adolescents aged 17 and 18, the researchers fitted a series of models that found support of the direct relationship linking emotional dysregulation with violent attitudes and behaviors.

OUR STUDY

The present study is an observational correlational research utilizing secondary data to investigate relationships among perceptual measures obtained from a sample of Saudi adolescent females. This design is appropriate given the purpose of the research, specifically the exploration of the magnitude and direction of the relationship between students' perceptions of their self-regulation and their attitudes toward violence. This makes the study cross-sectional, examining one sample at a single point in time. While such a design is weaker in comparison to longitudinal or experimental research, data on students' perceptions of self-regulation and violence is limited.

The sample utilized for the analysis in the present research is comprised of 132 girls, ages 10-15, attending Saudi schools. This group was part of a random sample of boys and girls utilized in previous research projects on parental attachment and school violence in the Kingdom. Data was collected under the auspices of the Saudi Department of Education and with proper consent of children's parents. The girls included in this research completed a series of questionnaires examining their perceptions on self-regulation and violence. Table 1 demonstrates the sample characteristics for the girls included in the analysis.

Table 1. Sample characteristics

Variable	Frequency	Percent
School Type		
Public	75	57.3
Private	56	42.7
Age		
10	7	5.3
11	25	18.9
12	18	13.6
13	22	16.7
14	32	24.2
15	28	21.2
Grade		
5th	22	16.7
6th	21	15.9
7th	25	18.9
8th	15	11.4
9th	49	37.1

The main independent variable in this study is self-regulation. It is operationalized through the Bandy and Moore (24) self-regulation scale. The questionnaire is comprised of 13 items. These measure three distinct sub-scales: emotional, behavioral, and cognitive self-regulation. The items are coded on a 4-value Likert-like metric. Reverse coding has been utilized to reflect higher score-equivalence for accurate agreement between the statements presented to participants. The main variable, composed of the score, is a total scale score of the 13 items (ranging from 13 to 52). Each sub-scale will then be used as a summated rating scale (4 items for behavioral regulation, 4 items for cognitive regulation, and five items for emotional regulation). Therefore, a respondent may receive a score between 4 and 16 on behavioral and cognitive regulations and between 5 to 20 on emotional regulation.

The main dependent variable for the study is students' perceptions of violence. To measure this construct, respondents completed the School

Survey on Violent Attitudes and Behaviors. The questionnaire measures the degree of violence perceived at the school by students and the actual violence experienced within the school in the month preceding the questionnaires' administration. A summated scale is ultimately constructed, using the first 8 items of the tool to exhibit perceptions of violence by the students. It modifies the original coding by placing a simple agreement or disagreement within the statement presented to the student. If the student agrees a score of 0 is given and if the student disagrees a score of 1 is assigned. This results in a scale ranging from 0 to 8, where higher scores reflect disagreement with violence. Therefore, one may understand that higher scores are reflections of peaceful means for solving conflicts. The questionnaires also included a number of control variables, including income. Income is measured on a scale of three categories: low = 1, medium = 2 and high = 3.

Correlational and regression methods are employed to test the magnitude and direction of relationships hypothesized in this research. Simple mean comparisons are also deployed in order to explore whether changes in one variable are associated with changes in another. Descriptive measures are also presented to aid the reader in understanding the degree to which Saudi girls perceive themselves to be self-regulated or inclined toward the use of violence to address their problems. Partial correlational analysis and multiple linear regression is finally utilized to test for the effect of income on the relationship between self-regulation and violent attitudes among Saudi adolescents.

FINDINGS

Perceptions of violence by Saudi adolescent females (N = 132) were demonstrated by a mean score of 3.96, indicating a moderate violent perception existing among girls in Saudi schools (the scale ranges between 0 and 8). The variation among girls is not very large given the standard deviation equivalence at 1.49. The score range was 1–7. Notice that the maximum observed score was 7 rather than 9, indicating that no student exhibited a fully non-violent agreement with the eight statements presented.

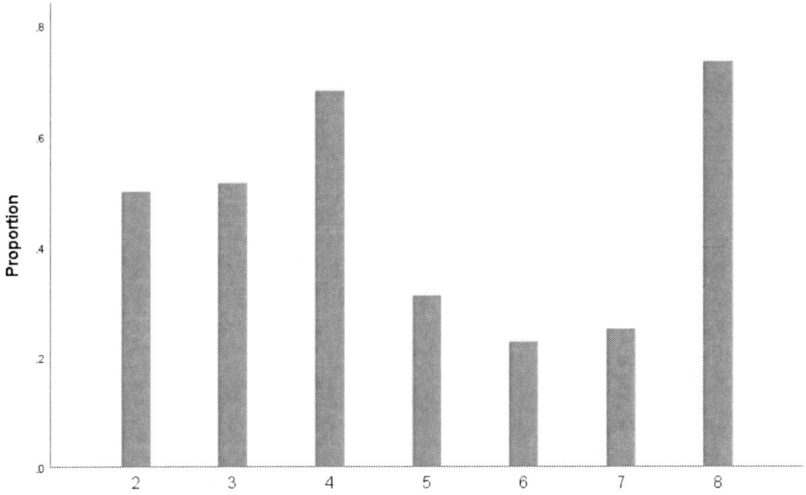

Figure 1. Saudi girls' perceptions of violent attitudes.

Figure 1 displays the proportions of agreement with items 2 thru 8 on the violent attitudes and behaviors survey. Note that higher proportions refer to disagreements with the violent descriptions in the items. Items 4 and 8 seem to receive the highest agreement among Saudi girls, indicating their agreement that "it is not ok to hit someone that hits you first" (item 8) and "violence creates more problems than it solves" (item 4). Saudi girls seem to agree more with the violent attitudes in items 5, 6, and 7. They would rather use violence to end problems (item 5), utilize violent means to handle problems compared to peaceful means (item 6), and employ violence to escape the coward or "chicken" descriptor arising from walking away (item 7).

Table 2. Saudi girls' self-regulation perceptions (N = 132)

Descriptive statistics					
	Range	Minimum	Maximum	Mean	*SD*
Self-regulation	35.00	11.00	46.00	33.9394	6.00224
Emotional regulation	13.00	3.00	16.00	10.8636	2.65805
Behavioral regulation	12.00	4.00	16.00	11.2652	2.96509
Cognitive regulation	12.00	4.00	16.00	11.8106	2.56855

Table 2 displays averages on a general measure self-regulation, emotional self-regulation, cognitive self-regulation, and behavioral self-regulation by Saudi girls. Self-regulation means are relatively low: 34 on a scale ranging between 13 and 52. Similarly, Saudi girls scored low on the subscales along the three dimensions comprising self-regulation (low on emotional self-regulation at 11 on a scale range between 5 and 20, and moderate on cognitive and behavioral self-regulations with an average of 11 on a scale range between 4 and 16 respectively).

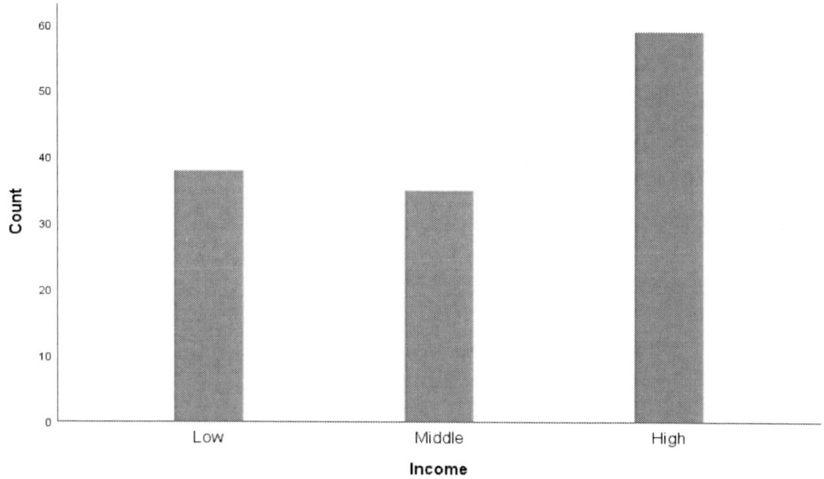

Figure 2. Perceptions of parental income.

Figure 2 displays the girls' perceptions of their parental income. It seems that the highest proportion reflect a relatively high income-perception among the participants. Further, the medium and low income-categories received similar frequencies from participants. This distribution may be due to the fact that many Saudi families prefer private schools (that are more expensive in comparison to public schools) where students may perceive themselves as being of higher income status given their attendance at such institutions.

Table 3 demonstrates the relationship between income level and violent attitudes among Saudi girls. It seems that variation in income does not induce large shifts in violence condoning by Saudi girls. Higher incomes seem to be associated with more violence conformity among the girls, while low income appears to carry the most desirable effect by increasing anti-violence attitudes among them. Nevertheless, such changes are not large practically, therefore one may exercise caution in concluding that such differences are of practical significance.

Table 3. Means comparison of income and violence

Violence			
Income	Mean	*N*	*SD*
Low	4.4474	38	1.44629
Middle	4.0000	35	1.41421
High	3.6271	59	1.50743
Total	3.9621	132	1.49506

Table 4. Mean comparison self-regulation and income level

Self-regulation			
Income	Mean	*N*	*SD*
Low	34.3421	38	7.02227
Middle	35.8571	35	4.99496
High	32.5424	59	5.56566
Total	33.9394	132	6.00224

Table 4 shows the distribution of self-regulation based on income level among Saudi girls. It is suggested that the averages of self-regulation do not shift significantly by variations within income levels. While this is true, it is also noticed that high income girls reported slightly lower levels of self-regulation. Similar to the earlier mean comparison, however, one needs to be careful in making sweeping generalizations given the small differences (3 points on a scale ranging from 13 to 52). This indicates that such miniscule variations do not warrant a conclusion of practical significance. A pattern also emerges in tables 5, 6, and 7, also demonstrating the changes in means between the different types of self-regulation and income.

Table 5. Mean comparison emotional regulation and income level

Emotional regulation			
Income	Mean	*N*	*SD*
Low	10.7895	38	3.12062
Middle	11.3714	35	2.25030
High	10.6102	59	2.55975
Total	10.8636	132	2.65805

Table 6. Mean comparison behavioral regulation and income level

Behavioral regulation			
Income	Mean	*N*	*SD*
Low	11.5526	38	2.71828
Middle	11.8000	35	2.72029
High	10.7627	59	3.21279
Total	11.2652	132	2.96509

Table 7. Mean comparison cognitive regulation and income level

Cognitive regulation			
Income	Mean	*N*	*SD*
Low	12.0000	38	2.97739
Middle	12.6857	35	1.99664
High	11.1695	59	2.45056
Total	11.8106	132	2.56855

Bivariate correlations were computed between income and self-regulation (r = -.147), income and violence perceptions (r = -.231), and self-regulation and violence perceptions (r = .424) among Saudi girls. It appears that there is a negative relationship between income level perceptions and attitudes against violence in schools. Higher income respondents seem to exhibit higher levels of violent attitudes. Meanwhile, the correlation between self-regulation and attitudes against violence is moderately positive (r = .42). The partial correlation between violence and self-regulation (controlling for income) investigated whether income levels change the relationship or not. The inclusion of income as a control has decreased the correlation from .42 to .406, a slightly yet not practically important decrease. One may conclude, based on such results, that there is a significantly moderate positive relationship between self-regulation and attitudes against violence held by Saudi girls. Levels of income do not appear to influence the strength or direction of such a relationship. Sixteen percent of variation in attitudes toward violence among Saudi girls can be explained by self-regulation alone.

Table 8. Regression

Variables	Beta	*T*	*p*-value
Income	-.172	-2.173	.032
Self-Regulation	.399	5.039	.000
R^2 0.210, N = 132			

Table 8 demonstrates the results of the multiple regression analysis, with violence attitudes as the dependent variable and self-regulation and income as independent variables. It appears that both independent variables are statistically significant with large t-statistics and small p-values. Further, the effect of self-regulation appears to supersede that of income. Betas represent changes in standard deviations in the dependent variable given a one unit increase in the standard deviation of the independent variable.

DISCUSSION

This study has uncovered low levels of self-regulation among Saudi girls, requiring immediate interventions to mitigate such a deficiency. Many solutions have been implemented in an attempt to improve self-regulation skills and abilities among adolescents. Perry-Parrish et al. (7) recommended the use of Mindfulness Based Cognitive Therapy to increase the awareness and attention span of adolescents dealing with uncomfortable situations. This type of therapy is designed to increase the focus of the adolescents on particular moments without any form of judgement or self-criticism before undergoing a series of exercises and techniques to improve their attention, focus, and concentration. The authors also suggested that the use of meditation along with such therapies have been shown to assist adolescents in enhancing self-control when faced with provocative situations.

The US Department of Health and Human Services has concluded that many current interventions for self-regulation in adolescence lack targeting and focus. Further, reports have suggested that existing programs do not heavily focus on instructing adolescents on how to manage distress, strong emotions, nor develop empathy. Therefore, more interventions that center the importance of preventing and controlling stress and developing stress coping skills need to be designed and implemented. Moreover, the inclusion of stakeholders within the community, including leaders, teachers, and mentors is an essential aspect of successful intervention to assist adolescents in coping with distress and self-regulation troubles.

While no official statistics exist on the number of Saudi girls who self-inflict harm to themselves due to difficulties in regulating their emotions, feelings, or thoughts, many interventions have been tried and proven successful in assisting patients improve in other contexts. Bjureberg et al. (25) reported significant improvements gained during an Individual Therapy for Adolescents treatment program where 17 girls were enrolled for 12 weeks. The treatment featured many exercises that increased the awareness and attention of the patients toward their emotions and self-control. Satisfaction with the treatment was high among the patients, and resulted in elevated completion rates. Further, the improvements in self-regulation during the period following the program has been recorded and observed as being high. Therefore, a need for the institution of individual therapy sessions or programs for special groups (such as girls self-inflicting harm) is necessary.

The use of creative therapies like art, music, or country-specific activities such as listening to the Quran in Saudi Arabia may carry a potential benefit for helping Saudi girls reduce stress and increase self-control. Dingle et al. (8) investigated the effect of a music listening program on self-regulation among two samples of adolescents (one at-risk and another without a particular psychological profile). Both samples reported improvements in the awareness, identification, and regulation of emotions once the program was completed. Participants also reported high satisfaction rates with the content and operation of the program. Smith-Israel (26) similarly investigated the effect of creative group therapy on adolescent anger management behaviors. He found that the program involving group work and activities decreased symptoms of emotional dysregulation and increased the tendency of students to seek help from teachers and mentors when faced with problems. The program was found to decrease the amount of disagreements and interruptions within the classroom, a typical measure of anger behavior among adolescents. Davis (27) also reached a similar conclusion when testing for the effect of art therapy om emotional regulation, with improvements in self-control being observed as a result of engaging in art therapy.

This study has also unearthed the tolerance deficit in Saudi schools. Violent attitudes appear to be rampant among adolescent Saudi females, giving rise to a wide range of potential academic, social, and behavioral problems such as bullying. One of the most important elements that decreases the degree of violence and aggression is the administration of Social and Emotional Learning programs. In the United States, The Collaborative on Academic, Social, and Emotional Learning (CASEL), blends elements of emotional intelligence and social relationships in order to build improvements in adolescents' awareness of their feelings and thoughts, thus enabling them to better control them. Similarly, in the United Kingdom, Social and Emotional Aspects Learning (SEAL) also targets students' skills in dealing with uncomfortable situations in schools. The observed effects of Social and Emotional Learning programs such as these have been decreased anger manifestations among adolescents and fostering of improved school climates where bullying is also decreased. Therefore, the Kingdom of Saudi Arabia should invest in such programs if it desires to curb violent attitudes and behaviors from its schools.

One proven strategy in curbing violent behaviors at schools is the provision of necessary professional development and training for teachers to cope with varying forms of violence. Studies have confirmed a negative relationship between further teacher preparation and violent incidents. Teachers who go through training in classroom management, behavioral control, and student motivation are more likely to have less episodes of violence. They are more likely to instruct students in self-regulation better than those who did not complete an equivalent training program. Saudi schools are lacking when it comes to specialized training on violent behavior and misconduct. Therefore, the ministry of education should prioritize the training of teachers in strategies that assist them in better management of the educational environment.

Most importantly, a holistic system of violence evaluation and monitoring should be implemented in Saudi educational institutions. Currently, these schools lack a comprehensive, systematic, and unified approach for assessing violent attitudes and behaviors among students. This hinders any realistic intervention given the limitations on accurate estimates of violence or any related feature such as emotional dysregulation. The system should be enforced at all schools (both private and public) and should be monitored from a special unit housed within the ministry of education. Data should be collected and analyzed so that interventions proposed to mitigate violent behaviors can be directly informed by facts rather than simply imposed on or by schools without any factual basis.

CONCLUSION

This analysis explored the association between self-regulation and aggressive attitudes among Saudi adolescent females (aged 11-15 years) by using a convenience sample of 132 participants from Jeddah. Results have confirmed earlier research findings by exhibiting support for the negative association found between self-regulation and aggressive attitudes and behaviors. Further, the study evaluated whether income moderates the relationship between self-regulation and aggression among Saudi girls. While higher income perceptions were associated with a slight increase in harboring aggressive attitudes, this difference did not warrant a conclusion of practical difference. Therefore, income has little to no effect on the relationship between self-regulation and aggression among Saudi adolescent females.

The findings also pointed to lower levels of self-regulation and moderate to high levels of aggressive attitude possession among Saudi girls. This necessitates immediate attention from educators and policy-makers in Saudi Arabia. Many established and innovative types of therapies have been attempted and proven successful in increasing levels of self-regulation and decreasing aggressive tendencies among adolescents across multiple contexts. Therefore, the Saudi government is urged to act through the implementation of counseling and therapy programs to target those girls with predetermined histories of psychopathologies.

This study has confirmed the robust association between self-regulation and violent propensities among adolescents. Such a relationship seems to be invariable with respect to sample, context, or country. This motivates the efforts, geared toward fostering better interventions that are compatible with local cultures, to increase levels of self-regulation across all of its dimensions. Most importantly, emotional regulation was shown as needing to be prioritized and presented as part of school curriculums through the social and emotional learning initiatives.

Lastly, this study marks one of the first systematic analyses of violent attitudes and tendencies among adolescent Saudi females. This issue is significant as the country is increasing in its diversity and educational opportunities for females alongside a liberal economy where women play a significant human resource role in constructing the modern Kingdom of Saudi Arabia. This makes focusing on the mental health needs of Saudi girls an essential area necessitating government and academic stakeholders to invest in. Little research or data has been available on the psychological well-being of Saudi women and girls, something this study seeks to alleviate and to bring about in the mainstream scholarship on psychology and education.

REFERENCES

[1] Perren S, Alsaker, F. Social behavior and peer relationships of victims, bully-victims, and bullies in kindergarten. J Child Psychol Psychiatry 2006;47:45-57.

[2] Hawker D, Boulton, M. Twenty years of research on peer victimization and psychosocial maladjustment: A meta-analytic review of cross-sectional studies. J Child Psychol Psychiatry 2000;41:441-55.

[3] Ryan W, Smith, D. Antibullying programs in schools: How effective are evaluation practices? Prev Sci 2009;10:248-60.

[4] AlBuhairan F, Tamim H, Al Dubayee M, AlDhukair S, Al Shehri S, Tamimi, W et al. Time for an adolescent health surveillance system in Saudi Arabia: Findings from "Jeeluna." J Adolesc Health 2015;57:263-9.

[5] Almuneef M, Qayad M, Aleissa M, Albuhairan F. Adverse childhood experiences, chronic diseases, and risky health behaviors in Saudi Arabian adults: A pilot study. Child Abuse Negl 2014;38:1787-93.

[6] Franken A, Moffitt T, Steglich C, Dijkstra J, Harakeh Z, Vollebergh W. The role of self-control and early adolescents' friendships in the development of externalizing behavior: The SNARE study. J Youth Adolesc 2016;45:1800-11.

[7] Perry-Parrish C, Copeland-Linder N, Webb L, Shields A, Sibinga E. Improving self-regulation in adolescents: current evidence for the role of mindfulness-based cognitive therapy. Adolesc Health Med Ther 2016;7:101-8.

[8] Dingle G, Hodges J, Kunde A. Tuned In emotion regulation program using music listening: Effectiveness for adolescents in educational settings. Front Psychol 2016;7:859.

[9] McLaughlin K, Hatzenbuehler M, Mennin D, Nolen-Hoeksema S. Emotion dysregulation and adolescent psychopathology: A prospective study. Behav Res Ther 2011;49:544-54.

[10] Zimmerman B. A social cognitive view of self-regulated academic learning. J Educ Psychol 1989;81:329.

[11] Heleniak C, King K, Monahan K, McLaughlin K. Disruptions in emotion regulation as a mechanism linking community violence exposure to adolescent internalizing problems. J Res Adolesc 2018;28:229-44.

[12] Bandura A. Social cognitive theory of self-regulation. Organ Behav Hum Decis Process 1991;50:248-87.

[13] DeWall C, Baumeister R, Stillman T, Gailliot M. Violence restrained: Effects of self-regulation and its depletion on aggression. J Exp Soc Psychol 2007;43:62-76.

[14] Tangney JP, Baumeister RF, Boone AL. High self-control predicts good adjustment, less pathology, better grades, and interpersonal success. J Pers 2004;72:271-324.

[15] Twenge JM, Zhang L, Im, C. It's beyond my control: A cross-temporal meta-analysis of increasing externality in locus of control, 1960-2002. Pers Social Psychol Rev 2004;8:308-19.

[16] Inzlicht M, Schmeichel B. What is ego depletion? Toward a mechanistic revision of the resource model of self-control. Perspect Psychol Sci 2012;7:450-63.

[17] Castillo R, Salguero J, Fernández-Berrocal P, Balluerka N. Effects of an emotional intelligence intervention on aggression and empathy among adolescents. J Adolesc 2013;36:883-92.

[18] Buss AH, Perry M. The Aggression Questionnaire. J Pers Soc Psychol 1992;63:452-9.

[19] Pérez-Albéniz A, De Paúl J, Etxebarría J, Montes MP, Torres E. Adaptación de Interpersonal Reactivity Index (IRI) al español [Spanish adaptation of the Interpersonal Reactivity Index]. Psicothema 2003;15:267-72.

[20] Özdemir Y, Vazsonyi A, Cok F. Parenting processes and aggression: The role of self-control among Turkish adolescents. J Adolesc 2013;36:65-77.

[21] Grasmick HG, Tittle CR, Bursik RJ, Arneklev BJ. Testing the core empirical implications of Gottfredson and Hirschi's general theory of crime. J Res Crime Delinq 1993;30:5-29.

[22] Watson M, Fischer K, Burdzovic Andreas J, Smith K. Pathways to aggression in children and adolescents. Harv Educ Rev 2004;74:404-30.

[23] Cuccì G, O'Leary K, Olivari M, Bonanomi A, Confalonieri E. Adolescent dating violence perpetration, emotion dysregulation, and parenting styles. J Fam Psychol 2019;33:12.

[24] Bandy T, Moore KA. Assessing self-regulation: A guide for out-of-school time program practitioners. Washington, DC: Child Trends, 2010.

[25] Bjureberg J, Sahlin H, Hellner C, Hedman-Lagerlöf E, Gratz K, Bjärehed J et al. Emotion regulation individual therapy for adolescents with nonsuicidal self-injury disorder: A feasibility study. BMC Psychiatry 2017;17:411.

[26] Smith-Israel S. Creative therapy and adolescents: Emotion regulation and recognition in a psycho-educational group for 9th grade students. Bachelor's thesis. Providence: RI: Providence College, 2009.

[27] Davis M. Heart in expression: An art therapy program for adolescents and the development of emotion regulation skill building. Dissertation. Chicago: IL: Adler University, 2014.

In: Pediatrics and Adolescent Health ISBN: 978-1-68507-490-6
Editors: J. Merrick and M. Morad

Chapter 12

FACTORS ASSOCIATED WITH SEXUAL ENGAGEMENT AMONG ADOLESCENTS IN SARAWAK, EAST MALAYSIA

Cheah Whye Lian[1], PhD, Halimah Awang[2,*], PhD, Chang Ching Thon[1], PhD, Low Wah Yun[3], PhD, Tong Wen Ting[3], MMedSc, Dev Nath Kaushal[1] and Hamizah Mohd Hassan[4]

[1]Faculty of Medicine and Health Sciences, Universiti Malaysia Sarawak, Sarawak
[2]Social Wellbeing Research Centre, Universiti Malaya, Kuala Lumpur, Malaysia
[3]Faculty of Medicine, Universiti Malaya, Kuala Lumpur, Malaysia
[4]National Population and Family Development Board, Ministry of Women, Family and Community Development, Kuala Lumpur, Malaysia

* Corresponding Author's E-mail: halima@um.edu.my.

ABSTRACT

This chapter examines the factors of sexual behaviours among schooling adolescents in Sarawak. Respondents for the study were adolescents aged 13 to 19 years from 16 secondary schools in Sarawak using self-administered questionnaire. Information on socio-demographic characteristics, knowledge on and attitudes towards sexual and reproductive health, involvement in risky lifestyle and sexual activities, family relationships, school attachment and religious beliefs were obtained. Chi-square tests and logistic regression analysis were performed to examine factors associated with sexual intercourse. A total of 1,462 students participated in the study, with 60.1% female respondents, mean age 15.6 ± 1.72 years old. The prevalence of sex engagement was 3.6%, majority aged 16-17 years (58.5%). Mean age at first sexual intercourse was 16.8 ± 1.27 years, with a minimum age of 14 years. Age of respondents, knowledge on SRH, risky behaviours, peers' risky behaviours, negative self-evaluation, cognitive inefficiency, perceived lack of motivation, religious belief and family support were significantly associated with sexual engagement. Logistic regression showed that age, respondents' risky behaviour and peers' involvement in sexual intercourse were significant risk factors of sexual engagement while a strong religious belief was a significant protective factor. Although the prevalence of sexual engagement was quite low compared to many other countries, there is a need to strengthen comprehensive sexual health education both at the school and community levels. It is important for adolescents to make informed decisions on their risky sexual behaviours as there are serious consequences of such behaviours on their current and future life.

INTRODUCTION

Adolescence is a period of self-discovery when young boys and girls experience biological, psychological, social and economic changes in their life. During this critical transition to develop self-regulatory capabilities, adolescents may resort to experimenting with a myriad of activities, whether beneficial or deleterious. They also have to undergo many challenges in order to attain a balance of social expectations and personal values. Due to their immaturity and inexperience, adolescents constantly place themselves at risk of undesired consequences of their decisions and actions especially so on matters related to sexual and reproductive health (SRH).

SRH as defined by World Health Organization is a state of complete physical, mental and social wellbeing, which includes the reproductive processes, function and system at all stages of life. It requires people to have a responsible, satisfying, positive, respectful and safe sex life, so that they have the capability to reproduce and freedom to decide if, when and how often to do so, without coercion, discrimination and violence (1). SRH development is an important aspect of adolescent health (2). However, in the past, adolescents' SRH had been overlooked resulting in an increase in the global burden of sexual ill health (3). As a consequence of unprotected sexual behaviours, there has been an increasing number of cases of sexually transmitted diseases, teenage pregnancy and unsafe abortions. In 2012, an estimated 2.1 million people aged 10 to 19 years from low- and middle-income countries were living with HIV (4) while the number of new HIV infections among young people aged 15-24 years reached 610,000 in 2016, of which 26,000 were aged 15-19 years (5). It was reported that approximately 16 million girls aged 15-19 in developing countries give birth each year, majority of them were unmarried (6) with some 3.9 million cases of unsafe abortions contributing to maternal mortality and other health problems (7). Maternal mortality was found to be a leading cause of death among young girls in Africa and South East Asia (8).

In Malaysia, although the prevalence of sexually transmitted human immunodeficiency viral (HIV) infection has declined from 2002 to 2010, it has been on an upward trend since then. At the end of 2014, a total of 3,517 new HIV cases were reported, signifying its importance as a public health issue (9). Within the new cases from 1990-2014, 34% were amongst young adults aged 13-29 years (9). What is more worrying is the rising incidence of sexual activity, unintended pregnancy and baby dumping? It was reported that sexual activity among adolescents aged 13-17 years increased from 2.3% in 2014 to 7.3% in 2017 and that 18,000 teenage girls become pregnant, unplanned, each year of which 50% end up in unsafe abortions (10). It should be noted that abortions are illegal in Malaysia except for situations where it would be life threatening for a pregnant woman to continue with her pregnancy, hence the alarming statistic of an average 100 baby dumping cases annually for more than a decade.

Data from the World Health Organization Global School-Based Student Health Survey 2012 indicated that 8.3% of students aged 12-17 years in Malaysia had ever had sex (11). A local study by (12) reported the prevalence of sexual activity among adolescents aged 18-19 was 6.4%, higher among males (8.9%) compared to females (3.6%). An earlier study conducted in 2012, among rural female adolescents found that 3.2% of them admitting their involvement in sexual activity in the past three months (13).

Adolescents' sexual behaviours are affected by many factors, ranging from biological, social, educational and psychological factors that can lead to high risk sexual behaviours such as sexual intercourse, unprotected sex and mouth-genital contact, early sexual debut, having multiple sex partners, having a high-risk partner, and having illegal abortion (14). In Malaysia there have been a number of studies on adolescents' sexual practices in recent years (11-12, 15-17). However, all of these studies were conducted in Peninsular Malaysia except for the study by (11) which analysed data for the whole country including Sarawak. There has not been any research focusing specifically on SRH among adolescents in Sarawak prior to the present study.

Sarawak located on the Borneo Island is the largest state of Malaysia. It has more than 40 sub-ethnic groups, each with distinct cultural background, Iban being the biggest ethnic group. The ethnic composition is very different from that of the whole country. Due to the complexity of cultural and religious practices, research on sexual issues is challenging and limited. According to the State Welfare, Women, and Community Wellbeing Minister of Sarawak, the number of teenage pregnancies has reduced, with 2,087 cases reported from January to October 2016 (18). However, Sarawak state statistics from 1989 to 2015 reported there were 2,178 HIV infections, and 480 of which resulted in AIDS-related deaths. Understanding the protective and risk factors of adolescents' involvement in sexual activity will help provide useful input for the development of strategies and programmes targeted at improving the overall sexual and reproductive health among young people. This research aimed to examine the prevalence of sexual engagement and the factors associated with it among adolescents in Sarawak so that specific interventions can be developed.

OUR STUDY

Data for the study were obtained from the National Population and Family Development Board (NPFDB) database. NPFDB commissioned this research in 2015 involving adolescents aged 13-19 years attending 16 public secondary schools in Sarawak in 2015. Data collection was through self-administered survey using structured questionnaire. Sample selection was based on multi-stage sampling procedure beginning with listing of all schools by region and district, taking into account the distribution of schools across urban, rural and various districts of the student population. Systematic sampling was used in the selection of schools based on the size of enrolment in relation to the total enrolment so that schools with large enrolment were more likely to be selected. Within each selected school, one class was randomly selected in each level of schooling, from Form 1 to Form 6 and all students in the selected class were included as potential respondents. Approval was obtained from the State Education Department and each of the selected schools while parental consent as well as informed consent from the students were obtained prior to the survey.

The questionnaire solicited among others information on socio-demographic characteristics, knowledge on and attitudes towards SRH related matters, respondents' involvement in risky sexual behaviours, friends' involvement in risky lifestyle and sexual activities, family relationships and school attachment. In addition, two questions on religious beliefs were included. Recognizing that young people's engagement in sexual risk behaviours is multifaceted and multifactorial, the study adopted the socio-ecological model which provided the framework for understanding the different influences including family, community and social environment and their relationships with one another (19). In order to develop effective interventions and policies, understanding of these factors is crucial.

Descriptive analysis was used to examine patterns of sexual engagement which was the variable of interest. Chi-square tests were performed to examine the associations between students' engagement in sex with selected independent variables followed by logistic regression analysis to assess the factors affecting their sexual engagement.

Table 1. Socio-demographic characteristics of respondents (N = 1,462)

Variable	Frequency (%)
Sex	
Male	583 (39.9)
Female	879 (60.1)
Ethnicity	
Iban	596 (40.8)
Malay	372 (25.4)
Bidayuh	183 (12.5)
Chinese	167 (11.5)
Others	144 (9.8)
Religion	
Christian	909 (62.2)
Islam	444 (30.4)
Buddha	96 (6.5)
Others	13 (0.9)
Current living arrangement	
Family	1,198 (81.9)
Hostel/Other	264 (18.1)
Parents' marital status	
Married	1,313 (89.8)
Divorced/separated/widowed	149 (10.2)
Locality	
Rural	1,175 (80.4)
Urban	287 (19.6)

Table 2. Associations between sexual engagement and respondents' socio-demographic and family background

Variable		**Respondents' engagement in sexual engagement**		
Overall		Yes	No	Chi-square, $\chi2$
		n (%)	n (%)	
		53 (3.6)	1409 (96.4)	
Gender	Male	29 (5.0)	554 (95.0)	4.98*
	Female	24 (2.7)	855 (97.3)	
Age (School) (years)	13-15	5 (0.7)	687 (99.3)	33.99**
	16-17	31 (5.6)	523 (94.4)	
	18 -19	17 (7.9)	199 (92.1)	
Time spent in a day without parents' supervision	<5 hrs	42 (3.3)	1243(96.7)	3.87*
	≥5 hrs	11 (6.2)	166 (93.8)	
Knowledge of SRH	High	29 (6.7)	406 (93.3)	16.40**
	Low	24 (2.3)	1003 (97.7)	
Attitude towards SRH	Positive	24 (2.6)	902 (97.4)	7.72**
	Negative	29 (5.4)	507 (94.6)	
Negative self-evaluation	High	31 (4.7)	622 (95.3)	4.25*
	Low	22 (2.7)	787 (97.3)	
Cognitive inefficiency	High	39 (4.6)	805 (95.4)	5.67*
	Low	14 (2.3)	604 (97.7)	
Perceived lack of motivation	High	35 (4.4)	756 (95.6)	3.15#
	Low	18 (2.7)	653 (97.3)	
The strength of my religious belief is the main barrier for me to have sex before legal marriage according to my religious practice	Agree	34 (3.0)	1098 (97.0)	5.55*
	Disagree	19 (5.8)	311 (94.2)	
Religious beliefs could not interfere with my basic right to have sexual relationship	Agree	18 (6.8)	246 (93.2)	9.40**
	Disagree	35 (2.9)	1163 (97.1)	
Family attachment	High	35 (2.9)	1157 (97.1)	8.77**
	Low	18 (6.7)	252 (93.3)	
Family involvement	High	38 (3.1)	1177 (96.9)	5.10*
	Low	15 (6.1)	232 (93.9)	

*p ≤ 0.05; **p ≤ 0.01.

FINDINGS

A total of 1,462 students (response rate of 95.9%) from 16 schools in both the urban and rural areas of Sarawak participated in the study, with 60.1% female respondents, mean age of 15.6±1.72 years. The ethnic distribution reflected the breakdown of the Sarawak population with Iban 40.8%, followed by Malay (25.4%), Bidayuh (12.5%), Chinese (11.5%) and 'others' (9.8%) which includes Melanau, Kenyah, Bisayah, Kayan, Kelabit, Penan and Indian. Christians comprised more than 60% followed by 30% Muslims and about 7% Buddhists. The majority of the respondents' parents were still married (89.8%) and they lived with their family (81.9%). In terms of locality, majority of the respondents were from rural schools (80.4%). Detailed information is presented in Table 1.

Sexual engagement

Of the total sample, 53 respondents (3.6%) admitted that they have had sex. The mean age at first sexual intercourse was 16.8 years with a standard deviation 1.27 years. Table 2 shows the associations between sexual engagement and the respondents' and family background characteristics which were statistically significant. Prevalence of sexual engagement was significantly higher among the boys than girls, among those who spent at least five hours without parents' supervision and increased with age. Significantly higher prevalence of sexual engagement was observed among respondents with high SRH knowledge, negative attitudes towards SRH, high negative self-evaluation, high cognitive inefficiency and high perceived lack of motivation compared with their respective counterparts. Expectedly, significantly lower prevalence of sexual engagement was found among respondents with strong religious beliefs and family support compared with their respective counterparts (see Table 2).

Table 3. Associations between sexual engagement and respondents' and peers' involvement in risky lifestyle behaviours

Variable		Respondents' engagement in sexual engagement		
Overall		Yes	No	χ^2
		n (%)	n (%)	
		53 (3.6)	1409 (96.4)	
Self - Drug	Yes	7 (14.3)	42 (85.7)	16.49**
	No	46 (3.3)	1367 (96.7)	
Self - Alcohol	Yes	31 (7.7)	373 (92.3)	26.19**
	No	22 (2.1)	1036 (97.9)	
Self - Smoking	Yes	23 (9.9)	210 (90.1)	30.95**
	No	30 (2.4)	1199 (97.6)	
Self - Dating	Yes	40 (8.0)	463 (92.0)	41.10**
	No	13 (1.4)	946 (98.6)	
Self - Clubbing	Yes	18 (17.3)	86 (82.7)	60.00**
	No	35 (2.6)	1323 (97.4)	
Self - Illegal racing	Yes	15 (10.8)	124 (89.2)	22.58**
	No	38 (2.9)	1285 (97.1)	
Self - Read/watch pornography	Yes	43 (8.8)	448 (91.2)	55.74**
	No	10 (1.0)	961 (99.0)	
Peer-Drug	Yes	11 (11.1)	88 (88.9)	17.03**
	No	42 (3.1)	1321 (96.9)	
Peer-Alcohol	Yes	25 (6.7)	350 (93.3)	13.36**
	No	28 (2.6)	1059 (97.4)	
Peer-Smoking	Yes	32 (7.3)	405 (92.7)	24.39**
	No	21 (2.0)	1004 (98.0)	
Peer-Sexual engagement	Yes	28 (25.9)	80 (74.1)	166.00**
	No	25 (1.8)	1329 (98.2)	
Peer-Pregnancy	Yes	9 (17.3)	43 (82.7)	28.89**
	No	44 (3.1)	1366 (96.9)	
Peer-Abortion	Yes	10 (22.7)	34 (77.3)	47.38**
	No	43 (3.0)	1375 (97.0)	

*$p \leq 0.05$; **$p \leq 0.01$.

The proportion of respondents who have had sex was significantly higher among those who were involved in risky lifestyle behaviours including drug, alcohol, smoking, dating, clubbing, illegal racing and read/watch pornography compared with respondents who were not involved in these activities. Similarly, prevalence of sexual engagement was significantly higher among respondents who have friends who were involved in risky lifestyle behaviours compared with those who did not have such friends (see Table 3).

Table 4. Logistic regression analysis of sexual engagement among school respondents

Variable		Coefficient	Standard error	Odds ratio
Age (years)	13-15	(reference)		
	16-17	1.399	0.551	4.051*
	18-19	1.010	0.613	2.747
The strength of my religious belief is the main barrier for me to have sex before legal marriage according to my religious practice	Disagree	(reference)		
	Agree	-1.046	0.388	0.351**
Self - Read/watch pornography	No	(reference)		
	Yes	1.250	0.447	3.489**
Self - Dating	No	(reference)		
	Yes	1.122	0.399	3.070**
Self - Clubbing	No	(reference)		
	Yes	1.356	0.510	3.880**
Peer-Sexual engagement	No	(reference)		
	Yes	2.336	0.458	10.340**

*$p \leq 0.05$; **$p \leq 0.01$.

Subsequently logistic regression was performed to examine the impact of all variables with significant Chi-square values on sexual engagement. The results in Table 4 indicates that age, the strength of religious belief, respondents' risky behaviours and peers' involvement in sex had significant influence on sexual engagement. Respondents aged 16-17 years were 4.1 times more likely to have had sex compared to those aged 13-15 years old. Similarly, respondents who read/watched pornographic materials, involved in dating, clubbing and, having friends who were involved in sexual engagement were 3.5 times, 3.1 times, 3.9 times and 10.3 times, respectively, more likely to have had sex compared to those who were not involved in such activities and not having friends who have had sex. The result also suggests that respondents who agreed that the strength of their religious belief was the main barrier for them to have sex before marriage were significantly less likely to engage in sex compared to those who did not agree (see Table 4).

DISCUSSION

The prevalence of sexual engagement of 3.6% among schooling adolescents is considered low compared with many developed countries and Southeast Asian countries studies (4.6% to 12.6%) (15, 20, 21). The reason could be due to the fact that the respondents were predominantly Muslims and Christians (more than 90%) which strictly speaking prohibit any sexual activity before marriage. Another reason could be because majority of the respondents were from rural schools which had limited access to information about sex and pornographic materials especially via the internet which in turn limits them from any experimentation of risky sexual behaviours.

In terms of mean age for the first sexual intercourse, this study reported 16.8 ± 1.27 years old, slightly older than the mean age of 14.9 ± 1.63 years found by (12) and that the proportion of respondents who have had sex increased with increasing age. This suggests that older adolescents could be more exposed to sex information and materials disseminated through media, internet and social network, which could influence them towards a more liberal attitude towards sexual engagement, often trigger their curiosity to experience sex related activities as they are also more susceptible to negative influence from peers (22, 23).

The literature showed that exposure to pornography, peer pressure, permissiveness regarding sexual engagement, and involvement in risk behaviour were the common significant contributing factors influencing sexual engagement among adolescents (12, 13). The association between involvement in risky behaviours and sexual engagement has been reported in past studies where frequent engagement in risky behaviours increased the tendency of engaging in sex, multiple sex partners and prostitution (13, 24).

Logistic regression showed that age, respondents' risk behaviours and their peers' involvement in sexual engagement were significant risk factors of sexual intercourse while the strength of religious belief was found to be a significant protective factor. Consistent with literature, engagement in risk behaviours such as reading and/or watching pornography, dating and clubbing as well as peers' risk behaviours increase the likelihood of sexual engagement among adolescents. Adolescence is the phase of growing up where young people transit from a family centred social environment to the outside world that encompasses peers (25). There is a range of risk behaviours that are commonly engaged by adolescents such as smoking, alcohol drinking, taking drugs, substance use and higher level of midnight activities that can lead to risky sexual behaviours (12-15, 21). Peers' risk behaviours can be one of the sources of pressure for adolescents to engage in sex related activities.

This study involved school-going adolescents in the state of Sarawak. This study is limited by the self-administered-questionnaire survey method as well as some sensitive questions that could possibly lead to response bias. The generalization of the findings is limited to school going adolescents. Non-school going adolescents such as those who dropped out may have had different experiences related to SRH.

Conclusion

Even though the prevalence of sexual engagement in this study was considered low, there is a need for interventions to reduce risk behaviours among adolescents as rural adolescents involving in their first sexual activity at a young age is still a cause for concern. The findings indicated the predictors of sexual engagement were age, respondents' risk behaviours and their peers' engagement in sex. There is a need to strengthen comprehensive sexual health education as well as the importance of religious belief both at the school and community levels to reach all adolescent age groups including those out of school. More efforts in the form of risk behaviour and health screening should be done by the primary care workers and physicians. Visits by the school health team lead by qualified primary care physicians should be frequent to create more awareness on SRH. Activities such as health promotion and intervention can be organized involving schools, parents and primary health care workers targeting at young adults. It is crucial that adolescents continued to be educated and guided until they attain healthy sexual development towards adulthood.

ACKNOWLEDGMENTS

Ethical approval for this study was obtained from the University of Malaya Medical Centre Medical Ethics Committee, 15th May 2013, and the Ministry of Education Malaysia, 20th August 2014. The study did not involve any human subject that would require informed consent. The authors would like to thank the National Population and Family Development Board for providing us with the data for purposes of analysis of this paper. The authors have no conflict of interest to declare. This project was commissioned to the University of Malaya Consultancy Unit by the National Population and Family Development Board, Ministry of Women, Family and Community Development, Malaysia (UPUM/SSC.147).

REFERENCES

[1] World Health Organization (WHO). Sexual and reproductive health. URL: www.who.int/reproductivehealth/en/.

[2] Morris JL, Rushwan H. Adolescent sexual and reproductive health: the global challenges. Int J Gynaecol Obstet 2015;131:40-2.

[3] Chandra-Mouli, V, Armstrong A, Amin A, Ferguson J. A pressing need to respond to the needs and sexual and reproductive health problems of adolescent girls living with HIV in low-and middle-income countries. J Int AIDS Soc 2015;18:20297.

[4] UNAIDS. Global Report: UNAIDS report on the global AIDS epidemic. Geneva: UNAIDS, 2013:2-106.

[5] UNICEF. Turning the tide against AIDS will require more concentrated focus on adolescents and young people. URL: https//data.unicef.org/topic/hivaids/adolescents-young-people/#.

[6] UNFPA. Girlhood, not motherhood: Preventing adolescent pregnancy. New York: UNFPA, 2015.

[7] Darroch J, Woong V, Bankole A, Ashford LS. Adding it up: costs and benefits of meeting the contraceptive need of adolescents. New York: Guttmacher Institute, 2016.

[8] Patton, GC, Coffey C, Cappa, C, Currie D, Riley L, Gore F, et al. Health of the world's adolescents: a synthesis of internationally comparable data. Lancet 2012;379:1665-75.

[9] Sha'ari N. Malaysia 2015 Country Responses To HIV/AIDS. Global aids response progress report Malaysia 2015. Kuala Lumpor: Ministry of Health Malaysia, 2015.

[10] The STAR Online. Plain facts on teenage pregnancy. URL: https://www.thestar.com.my/opinion/letters/2019/07/12/plain-facts-on-teenage-pregnancy.

[11] Ahmad N, Awaluddin SM, Ismail H, Samad R, Nik Abd Rashid, N. Sexual activity among Malaysian school-going adolescents: what are the risk and protective factors? Asia Pac J Public Health 2014;26:44-52.

[12] Awaluddin, SM, Ahmad NA, Saleh NM, Aris T, Kasim NM, Sapri NAM, et al. Prevalence of sexual activity in older Malaysian adolescents and associated factors. J Public Health Aspects 2015. http://dx.doi.org/10.7243/2055-7205-2-1.

[13] Ahmadian M, Hamsan HH, Abdullah H, Samah AA, Noor AM. Risky sexual behavior among rural female adolescents in Malaysia: a limited role of protective factors. Global J Health Sci 2014;6:165.

[14] Lee RLT, Yuen Loke A, Hung TTM, Sobel H. A systematic review on identifying risk factors associated with early sexual debut and coerced sex among adolescents and young people in communities. J Clinical Nurs 2018; 27:478-501.

[15] Lee, LK, Chen, PC, Lee, KK, Kaur, J. Menstruation among adolescent girls in Malaysia: a cross-sectional school survey. Singapore Med J 2006;47:869-74.

[16] National Population and Family Development Board. A study on risk and protective factors affecting adolescents' sexual and reproductive health in Peninsular Malaysia. Unpublished report, 2013.

[17] Nawi, AM, Roslan D, Idris IB, Hod R. Bullying and truancy: predictors to sexual practices among school-going adolescents in Malaysia: A cross-sectional study. Med J Malaysia 2017;72:298-305.

[18] Goh PP. Teen pregnancy cases on downtrend in Sarawak, this year at 2,087, says state Women's Minister. New Straits Times 2016 URL: http://www.nst.com.my/news/2016/11/192511.

[19] Henrich CC, Brookmeyer KA, Shrier LA, Shahar G. Supportive relationships and sexual risk behavior in adolescence: an ecological–transactional approach. J Pediatr Psychol 2005;31:286-97.

[20] Anwar M, Sulaiman SAS, Ahmadi K, Khan TM. Awareness of school students on sexually transmitted infections (STIs) and their sexual behavior: A cross-sectional study conducted in Pulau Pinang, Malaysia. BMC Public Health 2010;10:47.

[21] Manaf MRA, Tahir MM, Sidi H, Midin M, Jaafar NRN, Das S, Malek AMA. Premarital sex and its predicting factors among Malaysian youths. Comprehensive Psychiatry 2014;55:82-8.

[22] Ghule M, Balaiah D, Joshi B. Attitude towards premarital sex among rural college youth in Maharashtra, India. Sex Culture 2007;11:1-17.

[23] Izugbara CO. Tasting the forbidden fruit: The social context of debut sexual encounters among young persons in a rural Nigerian community. Aft J Reprod Health 2001;8:96-107.

[24] Peltzer K, Pengpid S. Prevalence and social correlates of sexual intercourse among school-going adolescents in Thailand. ScientificWorldJournal 2011; 11:1812-20.

[25] Stanton B, Li X, Pack R, Cottrell L, Harris C, Burns JM. Longitudinal influence of perceptions of peer and parental factors on African American adolescent risk involvement. J Urban Health 2002;79:536-48.

In: Pediatrics and Adolescent Health ISBN: 978-1-68507-490-6
Editors: J. Merrick and M. Morad

Chapter 13

EFFECT OF PEER AND PARENT-LED EDUCATIONAL INTERVENTION ON HIV KNOWLEDGE AND ATTITUDE OF IN-SCHOOL ADOLESCENTS IN SELECTED SECONDARY SCHOOLS IN OGUN STATE, NIGERIA

Olanrewaju Motunrayo Funmilayo, DrPH and Elebiju Oluwatoyin Juliana*
Department of Public and Allied Health,
Babcock University, Ilishan Remo,
Ogun State, Nigeria

ABSTRACT

HIV/AIDS is one of the world's greatest challenges for decades with sub-Saharan Africa bearing the greatest burden of the disease. Nigeria has the second largest number of people living with HIV/AIDS in sub-

* Corresponding Author's E-mail: elebiju2008@gmail.com.

Saharan Africa and has become a significant public health problem. AIDS is the leading cause of death among adolescents in Africa with 85% living in developing countries. Ogun state had a prevalence of 0.6% in year 2012 but increased to 1.6% in 2018. The main objective was to assess the effect of peer and parent-led educational intervention on HIV prevention among in-school adolescents in selected secondary schools in Ogun state Nigeria. The study population was selected in-school adolescents. The study utilized a quasi-experimental design. The multistage sampling technique was used in selecting participants. The mean age of adolescents was 14.90 ± 1.836. Less than 10% had a high level of knowledge and attitude of HIV/AIDS. The change in level of knowledge of adolescents between baseline and 8-weeks follow-up indicated a mean difference of 5.673, 7.945, 9.236 and -0.709 for the peer-led, parent-led, peer and parent-led and control groups. The interventions effected some changes in attitude of adolescents between baseline and 8-weeks follow-up. There was a mean difference of 5.800 ($p < 0.01$) among the adolescents in peer-led group, 10.200 ($p < 0.01$) in parent-led intervention group, 8.200 ($p < 0.01$) in peer and parent-led intervention group and a reduction in mean in control group (-3.164; $p < 0.01$). In conclusion, parent-led intervention had a higher impact on adolescents' knowledge and attitude compared to the other intervention.

INTRODUCTION

Human immunodeficiency virus infection and acquired immune deficiency syndrome (HIV/AIDS) have been one of the world's greatest challenges for decades with the sub-Saharan Africa bearing the greatest disease burden (1). Nigeria has the second largest number of people living with HIV/AIDS after South Africa in sub-Saharan Africa and the disease has become a significant public health problem. AIDS is the leading cause of death among young people in Africa and amounts to 85 percent living in developing countries (2). Globally, Africa has remained the most affected region by the epidemic recording over 67% of all people living with HIV globally and nearly three quarters (67%) of AIDS related deaths and over 50% of all HIV cases globally are young people (10-24 years) (3). Sub-Saharan Africa accounts for 9 out of 10 adolescent AIDS-related deaths and Africa's youth bulge may worsen the situation if immediate action is not taken (4).

Amongst the five countries with the highest burden of adolescent HIV; South Africa, Nigeria, Kenya, Tanzania and Uganda, only Nigeria is still experiencing an increase in young adolescent deaths. In Kenya, young adolescent deaths have reduced to half since peaking in 2007 and South Africa has seen a reduction of 17% since 2012 (5). Older adolescent deaths continue to increase particularly in South Africa and Nigeria. Comprehensive and accurate knowledge of HIV measured by the UN General Assembly on AIDS (UNGASS) knowledge indicator as percentage of young people aged 15–24 who both correctly identify ways of preventing the sexual transmission of HIV and who reject major misconceptions about HIV transmission is essential for behavior change (6). There is mounting evidence of the correlation between increased comprehensive knowledge and reduction in HIV incidence and prevalence in regions characterized by high HIV prevalence. Globally, evidence has shown that despite the high level of awareness of HIV among the youths, comprehensive knowledge of HIV remains unacceptably low, even in countries most affected by the epidemic (7).

Adolescents represent a growing share of people living with HIV worldwide. The number of adolescents dying from HIV related illnesses is estimated to have tripled over the last two decades; an estimated 1.9 million people are living with HIV in Nigeria accounting for a prevalence of 1.4%. Among children aged 0–14 years, HIV prevalence is estimated to be 0.2% (7). The HIV prevalence of adolescents in Nigeria is estimated to be 3.5%, the highest among countries in West and Central Africa (8). West and Central Africa accounts for 6 per cent of the global population, but has the second largest which is likely to increase because of high HIV incidence among adolescents. It has been reported that in societies where HIV prevalence is high, economic growth rates have been reduced, life expectancy has been cut short, rate of mortality increased, poverty level deepened, number of orphans multiplied, business activities shrank, level of investment declined, public and private health expenditures increased, human resources destroyed, industry and agricultural sustainability hampered while household income level reduced (9). A survey reported that evidently, the effect of the disease on growth through its impact on life expectancy overwhelmingly remained negative (10). Ogun state had a prevalence of 0.6% in the year 2012 (11), but current result revealed the prevalence has increased to 1.6% (12).

The main objective of the study was to assess the effect of peer and parent-led educational intervention on HIV prevention among in-school adolescents in selected secondary schools in Ogun state Nigeria.

OUR STUDY

The study utilized a quasi-experimental design comprising of three experimental group and one control group in order to assess the effect of peer-led educational intervention on HIV knowledge and attitude of in-school adolescents in selected secondary schools in Ogun State, Nigeria. The multistage sampling technique was used in selecting the participants. A senatorial district in Ogun state was selected by simple random sampling through balloting; and from the senatorial district selected; one local government were randomly selected. The list of secondary schools was obtained from the Ministry of Education and one public secondary school was randomly selected from the selected local government area. Upon selection of the secondary schools, the students were randomly selected from each of one junior class (JSS3); this is because the least age to be in JSS3 is 10 years so this made them eligible for the study and the three (3) senior classes (SS1, SS2 and SS3) through random sampling. The peer educator was randomly selected from the student leaders of the school. The peer educators were trained for a week after which they were evaluated.

The study population was in-school adolescents in selected government secondary schools in Ogun State. The students were within the age range of 10 and 19 years old from the selected schools. The criteria were the adolescents chosen were fully registered students in the selected secondary schools. The students were between the ages of 10 – 19 years old and were selected with the assumption that they are registered students in the school for the duration of the study intervention. They were approached for their willingness to consent to participate in the study. The exclusion criteria for participants in this study are, Students who were not fully registered at the time of the study; Adolescents who were not attending the selected school; Teaching and non-teaching staff members of institution were excluded from the study and The students above and below the age bracket of young adulthood (10-19 years) were excluded from this study.

The sample size was derived from the computation using a level of significance of 95% and 80% power. The prevalence rate of HIV in Ogun state is 1.6. Thus, the sample size was determined using the given prevalence:

$$N = \frac{(Z_\alpha + Z_\beta)^2 \text{ X } P_0 (1 - P_0)}{(D)^2}$$

N = Sample size

Z_α = Standard normal deviation at 95% confidence interval (1.96)

Z_β = Statistical power at 80% confidence interval; 0.84

P_0 = prevalence at 50%

P_1 = 80% (desired level of outcome variable)

d = level of precision at 5%

$$n = \frac{(1.96 + 0.84)^2 \times 0.016(1 - 0.016)}{(0.05)^2}$$

$$\frac{(2.8)^2 \times 0.016(0.984)}{(0.05)^2}$$

$$\frac{0.12343296}{0.0025}$$

$$= 49.37 \simeq 50$$

The minimum sample size was 50. 10% of the minimum sample size was added to take care of attrition. The total number of participants after adding 10% of 50 was = 50 + 5 $\simeq$ 55, so approximately 55 participants per group was considered for the study. Based on the computation a total number of 220 participants from the two selected secondary schools were enrolled for this study (representing 55 people per group).

A quantitative approach was adopted for the study. Instrument was developed using information gathered from review of literature and instruments from other similar studies. The instrument was a semi-structured, participant-administered questionnaire, which solicited information on the demographic characteristics; knowledge and attitude of In-School Adolescents in Selected Secondary Schools in Ogun State, Nigeria. The same instrument was administered at baseline; immediate post intervention and 8-weeks follow up. The instrument is sectioned as follows:

- Section A: This aimed at assessing respondents' socio demographic factors which include their gender, age, religion, class and ethnicity.
- Section B: This aimed at assessing participants' knowledge of HIV, which consisted of thirty-two dichotomous questions of Yes/No, that was measured on a 32-point rating scale
- Section C: This section evaluated participants' attitudinal disposition towards HIV prevention; this was measured on a 42-point Likert scale of Strongly Agree (SA), Agree (A), Disagree (D) and Strongly Disagree (SD).

To ascertain the reliability of the instrument, a test retest was conducted for internal consistency of the instrument using 10% of the projected sample size. The instrument was distributed to 10 adolescents in a community with same characteristics as the study population. The reliability score generated was 0.723. This study seeked ethical approval from the ethical committee of the university – Babcock University Health Research and Ethics Committee (BUHREC); the Ministry of Health Research Ethics and Ministry of Education Planning Research and Statistics, Ogun State for ethical approval to conduct the study. All persons was informed that their participation is voluntary and inform consent was sought from all participants prior to their participation. Confidentiality of participants was maintained as no personal identifying information will be collected on the questionnaire.

Data analysis

The data collected for the study was collated, entered and coded using the statistical package for social sciences (SPSS), version 23. Both descriptive and inferential statistics was used for data analysis. Results are presented with frequency counts, percentages was used for descriptive statistics and the statistical level of significance for the inferential statistics will be set at $p \leq 0.05$. Means and standard deviations was computed for items within groups. The socio-demographic variables were tested for randomization between the four groups. Hypothesis was tested using inferential statistics such as Pearson Product Moment Correlation, T-test for Independent Samples and Multiple Regression Analysis. Chi-square will be used to determine association between categorical variables; T-test to compare means of continuous variables, Repeated measure ANOVA to test pairwise, within and between variable comparison.

FINDINGS

There were more students in the middle adolescence (14-16 years) age bracket across the three intervention and control groups. The mean age of the students was between 14.5 years and 15 years across the four groups. In each of the groups, over half of all the students were females (see Table 1). The adolescents were recruited from the junior secondary school class 3 and senior secondary school classes 1 to 3 (see Table 2). Majority of the students were Christians and only a small combined proportion reported to be traditionalists. The ethnic distribution showed that majority of the students were from the Yoruba ethnic group and a few from the Igbo, Hausa and other minority ethnic tribes (see Table 2).

Table 1. Baseline distribution of socio-demographic characteristics of respondents in control and intervention groups: Age and gender

Variables	Peer-led Group N (%)	Parent-led Group N (%)	Peer and Parent-led Group N (%)	Control N (%)	p-value
Age					
10 – 13	9 (16.4)	9 (16.4)	9 (16.4)	19 (32.7)	
14 – 16	37 (67.3)	38 (69.1)	38 (69.1)	22 (40.0)	0.883[a]
17 - 19	9 (16.4)	8 (14.5)	8 (14.5)	15 (27.3)	
Total	55 (100)	55 (100)	55 (100)	55 (100)	
Mean ± SD	14.89 ± 1.583	14.96 ± 1.360	14.85 ± 1.919	14.87 ± 2.373	
Gender					
Male	12 (21.8)	26 (47.3)	22 (40.0)	20 (36.4)	
Female	43 (78.2)	29 (52.7)	33 (60.0)	35 (63.6)	0.212[b]
Total	55 (100)	55 (100)	55 (100)	55 (100)	

[a]p-value obtained by T-test. [b]p-value obtained by Chi-Square. *significant at < 0.05.

Table 2. Baseline distribution of socio-demographic characteristics of respondents in control and intervention groups: Class, religion and ethnicity

Variables	Peer-led Group N (%)	Parent-led Group N (%)	Peer and Parent-led Group N (%)	Control N (%)	p-value
Class					
JSS 3	18 (32.7)	21 (38.2)	27 (49.1)	20 (36.4)	
SS 1	14 (25.5)	12 (21.8)	16 (29.1)	9 (16.4)	
SS 2	12 (21.8)	13 (23.6)	8 (14.5)	12 (21.8)	0.810a
SS 3	11 (20.0)	9 (16.4)	4 (7.3)	14 (25.5)	
Total	55 (100)	55 (100)	55 (100)	55 (100)	
Religion					
Christianity	44 (80.0)	37 (67.3)	41 (74.5)	49 (89.1)	
Islam	8 (14,5(	18 (32,7)	12 (21.8)	5 (9.1)	0.160a
Traditional	3 (5.5)	0 (0.0)	2 (3.6)	1 (1.8)	
Total	55 (100)	55 (100)	55 (100)	55 (100)	
Ethnicity					
Yoruba	41 (74.5)	46 (83.6)	40 (72.7)	49 (89.1)	
Igbo	6 (10/9)	5 (9.1)	0 (0.0)	4 (7.3)	
Hausa	0 (0.0)	1 (1.8)	0 (0.0)	0 (0.0)	0.375a
Others	8 (14.5)	3 (5.5)	15 (27.3)	2 (3.6)	
Total	55 (100)	55 (100)	55 (100)	55 (100)	

[a]p-value obtained by Chi-Square. *significant at < 0.05.

Baseline comparison of the socio-demographic characteristics of the respondents among the groups (intervention groups 1, 2 3 and control group)

There were more students in the middle adolescence (14-16 years) age bracket across the three intervention and control groups. The mean age of the students was between 14.5 years and 15 years across the four groups. In each of the groups, over half of all the students were females (see Table 1). The adolescents were recruited from the junior secondary school class 3 and senior secondary school classes 1 to 3 (see Table 2). The majority of the students were Christians and only a small combined proportion reported to be traditionalists. The ethnic distribution showed that majority of the students were from the Yoruba ethnic group and a few from the Igbo, Hausa and other minority ethnic tribes (see Table 2). Hence, the respondents in the four groups had similar socio-demographic characteristics and their selection into the study was randomized.

Table 3. Baseline distribution of adolescents' awareness of HIV/AIDS

Variables	Peer-led Group N (%)	Parent-led Group N (%)	Peer and Parent-led Group N (%)	Control N (%)	p-value
Ever heard about HIV/AIDS					
Yes	55 (100)	55 (100)	55 (100)	55 (100)	
No	0 (0.0)	0 (0.0)	0 (0.0)	0 (0.0)	
Total	55 (100)	55 (100)	55 (100)	55(100)	
Source of Information					0.378a
Friends	12 (21.8)	14 (25.5)	10 (18.2)	22 (40.0)	
Parents	27 (49.1)	14 (25.5)	22 (40.0)	21 (38.2)	
Newspaper	1 (1.8)	2 (3.6)	1 (1.8)	2 (3.6)	
Textbooks	4 (7.3)	11 (20.0)	3 (5.5)	2 (3.6)	
Radio	6 (10.9)	7 (12.7)	8 (14.5)	2 (3.6)	
Internet	0 (0.0)	2 (3.6)	4 (7.3)	1 (1.8)	
Television	2 (3.6)	4 (7.3)	2 (3.6)	5 (9.1)	
Flyers	3 (5.5)	1 (1.8)	5 (9.1)	0 (0.0)	

Table 3. (Continued)

Variables	Peer-led Group N (%)	Parent-led Group N (%)	Peer and Parent-led Group N (%)	Control N (%)	p-value
Total	55 (100)	55 (100)	55 (100)	55 (100)	
Ever sought information on HIV/AIDS					
Yes	53 (96.4)	54 (98.2)	54 (98.2)	53 (96.4)	0.877a
No	2 (3.6)	1 (1.8)	1 (1.8)	2 (3.6)	
Total	55 (100)	55 (100)	55 (100)	55 (100)	
Where did you obtain such information?					0.093a
Library	5 (9.1)	4 (7.3)	4 (7.3)	1 (1,8)	
School	31 (56.4)	24 (43.6)	33 (60.0)	35 (63.6)	
Health center/Hospital	6 (10.9)	10 (18.2)	3 (5.5)	16 (29.1)	
Textbooks	5 (9.1)	13 (23.6)	9 (16.4)	3 (5.5)	
Parents	3 (5.5)	4 (7.3)	4 (7.3)	0 (0.0)	
Others	5 (9.1)	0 (0.0)	2 (3.6)	0 (0.0)	
Total	55 (100)	55 (100)	55 (100)	55 (100)	

[a]p-value obtained by Chi-Square. *significant at < 0.05.

Baseline distribution of adolescents' awareness of HIV/AIDS

At baseline, all the participants across the three intervention and control groups reported that they had heard about HIV/AIDS. In the peer-led intervention group, almost half of the students reported to have obtained their information from their parents; half got their information from both friends and parents in the parent-led intervention group; about 40% of the students in the parent and peer-led and control group got their information from their parents (see Table 3). Over 95% of all students across the four groups reported to have individually sought information about HI/AIDS at some period and the preferred source of information for the adolescents was in their schools.

Table 4. Change in knowledge in the peer-led intervention group, parent-led intervention group, peer and parent led intervention group and control group

Variables	Peer-led Group N (%)	Parent-led Group N (%)	Peer and Parent-led Group N (%)	Control N (%)
Baseline				
Low (0 – 8)	2 (3.6)	4 (7.3)	14 (25.5)	16 (29.1)
Moderate (9 – 16)	49 (89.1)	50 (90.9)	36 (65.5)	36 (65.5)
High (17 – 24)	4 (7.3)	1 (1.8)	5 (9.1)	3 (5.5)
Total	55 (100)	55 (100)	55 (100)	55 (100)
Mean ± SD	13.11 ± 2.386	12.11 ± 2.529	11.0 ± 3.477	10.42 ± 3.430
Post Intervention				
Low (0 – 8)	0 (0.0)	0 (0.0)	0 (0.0)	6 (10.9)
Moderate (9 – 16)	27 (49.1)	13 (23.6)	19 (34.5)	43 (78.2)
High (17 – 24)	28 (50.9)	42 (76.4)	36 (65.5)	6 (10.9)
Total	55 (100)	55 (100)	55 (100)	55 (100)
Mean ± SD	16.47 ± 2.456	18.55 ± 2.537	17.62 ± 2.528	12.09 ± 3.351
8-weeks Follow Up				
Low (0 – 8)	0 (0.0)	0 (0.0)	0 (0.0)	21 (38.2)
Moderate (9 – 16)	7 (12.7)	1 (1.8)	1 (1.8)	33 (60.0)
High (17 – 24)	48 (87.3)	54 (98.2)	54 (98.2)	1 (1.8)
Total	55 (100)	55 (100)	55 (100)	55 (100)
Mean ± SD	18.78 ± 1.883	20.05 ± 1.533	20.29 ± 1.449	9.71 ± 3.270
Effect size	0.851	0.911	0.871	0.532
Mean difference (Baseline to follow up)	5.673	7.945	9.236	-0.709

Baseline distribution of adolescents' knowledge and attitude of HIV/AIDS

The knowledge of the adolescents on information regarding HIV/AIDS such as transmission routes, risks and causes was measured with a 23-item scale. The responses were grouped on a scale and the results showed that majority of the adolescents in the peer-led and parent led intervention groups had a moderate level of knowledge regarding HIV/AIDS while about two-thirds of the participants from the peer and parent-led and control groups had a moderate level of knowledge. Across the four groups, less than 10% of the participants had a high level of knowledge of HIV/AIDS with only one person in the parent-led intervention group (see Table 4).

The level of attitude of the participants was measured with a 10-item scale. The results showed that 56.4%, 43.6%, 40.0% and 76.4% of the adolescents had a positive attitude towards HIV/AIDS (see Table 5).

Table 5. Change in attitude in the peer-led intervention group, parent-led intervention group, peer and parent led intervention group and control group

Attitude	Peer-led Group N (%)	Parent-led Group N (%)	Peer and Parent-led Group N (%)	Control N (%)
Baseline				
Negative (0 15) Positive (16 – 30)	24 (43.5) 31 (56.4)	31 (56.4) 24 (43.6)	33 (60.0) 22 (40.0)	13 (23.6) 42 (76.4)
Total	55 (100)	55 (100)	55 (100)	55 (100)
Mean ± SD	16.11 ± 4.246	14.64 ± 3.262	13.96 ± 4.933	17.27 ± 5.020
Post Intervention				
Negative (0 15) Positive (16 – 30)	5 (9.1) 50 (90.9)	2 (3.6) 53 (96.4)	4 (7.3) 51 (92.7)	31 (56.4) 24 (43.6)
Total	55 (100)	55 (100)	55 (100)	55 (100)
Mean ± SD	20.27 ± 3.325	22.07 ± 3.641	20.93 ± 4.476	14.82 ± 4.355
8-weeks Follow Up				
Negative (0 15) Positive (16 – 30)	1 (1.8) 54 (98.2)	1 (1.8) 54 (98.2)	0 (0.0) 55 (100.0)	31 (56.4) 24 (43.6)
Total	55 (100)	55 (100)	55 (100)	55 (100)
Mean ± SD	21.94 ± 3.233	24.84 ± 3.500	22.16 ± 3.219	14.11 ± 3.971
Effect size	0.649	0.852	0.719	0.651
Mean Differences (Baseline to follow up)	5.800	10.200	8.200	-3.164

Effectiveness of educational intervention on adolescents' knowledge of HIV

This section addresses the effectiveness of the intervention modules (peer-led education, parent-led education and peer and parent-led education) on the level of knowledge of adolescents. The majority of adolescents in the peer-led and parent-led groups had a moderate level of knowledge. At post intervention, all adolescents in the intervention groups were either in the moderate or high-level category of knowledge. At 8-weeks follow up, the proportion of the adolescents who recorded a moderate level of knowledge in all intervention groups had dropped. The mean of the adolescents' level of knowledge had increased (see Table 4).

Change in HIV knowledge from baseline to 8-weeks follow-up

The change in the level of knowledge of the adolescents between the baseline and the 8-weeks follow up indicated a mean differences of 5.673, 7.945, 9.236 and -0.709 for the peer-led intervention, parent-led intervention, peer and parent-led intervention and control groups respectively (see Table 4). The observed difference in means in all the four groups across these periods was statistically significant ($p < 0.01$). The result indicates that the peer and parent-led intervention had a greater effect on the change in knowledge between the baseline and 8-weeks follow up periods.

Effectiveness of educational intervention on adolescents' attitude towards HIV

The effectiveness of the educational interventions was measured by computing the mean differences for the periods through the groups. The adolescents in the control group had the highest mean ± SD (17.27 ±

5.020) at baseline among the four groups. However, at post intervention, there was an increase in the mean ± SD for the intervention groups (see Table 5) and a decrease in the control group.

Change in attitude towards HIV from baseline to 8-weeks follow-up

The interventions effected some changes in the attitude of the adolescents between the baseline and the 8-weeks follow up period. There was a mean difference of 5.800 ($p < 0.01$) among the adolescents in the peer-led group, 10.200 ($p < 0.01$) in the parent-led intervention group, 8.200 ($p < 0.01$) in the peer and parent-led intervention group and a reduction in mean in the control group (-3.164; $p < 0.01$) (see Table 5). During this period, the parent-led intervention group had a higher impact on the adolescents' attitudinal disposition compared to the other intervention modules.

Test of hypothesis

Two hypotheses were tested in this study to determine the effect of the intervention programs on the HIV prevention skills of the adolescents in Ogun State. The decision rule applied stated that a p-value less or equal to 0.05 would have the null hypothesis rejected.

Research hypothesis 1

There will be no difference between the levels of knowledge of HIV prevention among adolescents at baseline and 8-weeks follow-up.

A paired T-test analysis was conducted to explore the difference in means of the adolescents' level of knowledge regarding HIV infection. The result of the t-test showed that the observed difference in mean in the peer-led group ($\Delta = 5.673$; $t_{54} = 17.015$; $p < 0.01$), parent-led group

($\Delta = 7.945$; $t_{54} = 23.454$; $p < 0.01$) and peer and parent-led group ($\Delta = 9.236$; $t_{54} = 19.026$) were statistically significant (see Table 6).

Table 6. Paired sample T-test showing the paired differences between the adolescents' level of knowledge at baseline and 8-weeks follow-up

Variable: Knowledge	N	Mean Diff	SE	df	t	Sig
Peer-led						
Baseline vs 8-weeks follow up	55	5.673	0.333	54	17.015	0.000a*
Parent-Led						
Baseline vs 8-weeks follow up	55	7.945	0.339	54	23.454	0.000a*
Peer and Parent-led						
Baseline vs 8-weeks follow up	55	9.236	0.485	54	19.026	0.000a*
Control						
Baseline vs 8-weeks follow up	55	0.709	0.109	54	6.500	0.000a*

[a]p-value obtained by t-test.
*significant at $p < 0.05$.

Table 7. Paired sample T-test showing the paired differences between the adolescents' attitudinal disposition towards HIV prevention at baseline and 8-weeks follow-up

Variable: Attitude	N	Mean Diff	SE	df	T	Sig
Peer-led						
Baseline vs 8-weeks follow up	55	5.800	0.664	54	8.730	0.000a*
Parent-Led						
Baseline vs 8-weeks follow up	55	10.200	0.595	54	17.148	0.000a*
Peer and Parent-led						
Baseline vs 8-weeks follow up	55	8.200	0.701	54	11.700	0.000a*
Control						
Baseline vs 8-weeks follow up	55	3.164	0.315	54	10.029	0.000a*

[a]p-value obtained by t-test.
*significant at $p < 0.05$.

The null hypothesis is rejected in favor of the alternative hypothesis. This implies that there is a difference as a result of the interventions on the level of knowledge of the adolescents in Ogun State.

Research hypothesis 2

There will be no significant difference between the levels of attitude towards HIV prevention of the adolescents at baseline and 8-weeks follow-up.

A paired T-test analysis was conducted to determine if the difference observed in the means of attitude of adolescents at baseline and 8-weeks follow up. The result showed that the observed difference in means in the peer-led group ($\Delta = 5.800$; $t_{54} = 8.730$; $p < 0.01$), parent-led group ($\Delta = 10.200$; $t_{54} = 17.148$; $p < 0.01$) and peer and parent-led group ($\Delta = 8.200$; $t_{54} = 11.700$) were statistically significant (see Table 7).

The result indicated that the null hypothesis is rejected in favor of the alternative hypothesis. This implies that the interventions affected a change in the attitudinal disposition of the adolescents in Ogun State towards HIV prevention.

CONCLUSION AND DISCUSSION

This section presents the discussion of study, which examined the effectiveness of peer and parent-led education programs on HIV prevention among adolescents in Ogun State, Nigeria. This discussion gives reasons for findings in the study as well as comparison with results from previous studies. The results from the study provide insight into the level of knowledge, attitudinal disposition, perception and self-efficacy to prevent HIV among adolescents in the study area. The participants were recruited secondary schools within the state. The response rate during the follow-up periods after the intervention was excellent. More of the participants were females compared to the proportion of males.

School-based HIV/AIDS prevention programmes play a significant role in HIV prevention. About 46% of Nigeria's population are young people under the age of 15 years who are at the core of their developmental period hence making schools a good platform to reach these young people. Previous studies have indicated that low levels of knowledge and misconceptions about the causes and prevention of HIV are widespread in Africa especially in the rural areas (13-15). This indicate that a large percentage of people have erroneous beliefs about the transmission routes of the virus. The level of awareness of the adolescents from this study was high and friends and parents were the sources of first information on HIV. Adolescents aged 15-19 years have been found to demonstrate high awareness of HIV/AIDS but some have been reported to be lacking in the aspect of specific knowledge of the disease (16). Similar to reports of cross-sectional studies conducted by Haddison et al. (17) and Nubed and Akoachere (18) in Cameroon, our respondents reported sexual education in school as the main sources of information on HIV/ AIDS. This implies that the school was a common source of HIV and AIDS information which augers well for school-based HIV and AIDS programs.

Acquisition of knowledge of HIV/AIDS may be a powerful weapon in the fight against the uprising epidemic. Individuals, especially sexually active adolescents who lack the knowledge and skills required to fight being infected by the virus are less equipped to protect themselves from the predisposing factors influencing the transmission and hence, the virus. The results of this study showed that the adolescents had a fairly moderate level of knowledge of HIV transmission and risks. In line with this, previous studies conducted among adolescents in Nigeria had established similar results (20-21). In the absence of a vaccine or cure, being aware of and protecting against the militating factors of HIV is of uttermost importance.

The educative intervention modules had an impact on the adolescents' level of knowledge on HIV prevention. There was a significant increase in the level of knowledge of HIV-related information after the intervention was administered and the increased knowledge persisted over a 4-week follow up period. The proportion of the adolescents who recorded a moderate level of knowledge in all intervention groups had dropped while the proportion of adolescents who had a high level had increased. The mean of the adolescents' level of knowledge had increased. This is evidence that education offered through different modules or channels and tailored to the need of adolescents will help improve understanding of the virus. Interventions are effective in changing misconceptions, misunderstandings and ideas about the HIV. Stonbraker et al. (21, and Kirby et al. (22), reported similar result; It is noteworthy that the parent-led intervention program had a higher effect size on the level of knowledge of adolescents on HIV prevention compared to the other modules. Implementation researches can help bridge the gaps in knowledge, attitude and practice levels. These levels can be increased in communities if there are adequate and evidence-based intervention administered to educate people about the necessary information. High levels of knowledge may have impact on the attitude and practice and eventually, people's behaviors (22). Attitude, which includes beliefs, ideas and emotional expressions serve as a predisposing factor to sexual risk behaviors, which in turn could cause HIV infections.

To investigate the attitudinal disposition of the adolescents at baseline, the students were asked questions, which assessed the nature of their attitudes towards HIV prevention. The results revealed that, overall, only 53% had a positive attitude towards HIV prevention. Similar to reports published by Choy et al. (23), there was a change in the level of attitudes of the adolescents the intervention induced a change in their attitudinal disposition and there was an observed participant had a better attitude towards HIV prevention and the effectiveness of the educative intervention which was tailor toward cognitive skills enhancement with a significant relationship. A comparison of the attitude scores across the intervention groups showed that contrary to my assumption, the parent-led intervention had a higher level of impact on the adolescent's attitudinal disposition.

Based on the results of this study, adolescents were able to develop better cognitive skills related to HIV prevention when they had a parent figure facilitating the program. Wamoyi et al. (24) pointed out that it is evidence that parent-child communication could be more effective in the reduction of new HIV infections among young people. Communication between parents and young people about sexuality issues especially those related to sexually transmitted infections including HIVAIDS, teenage pregnancy, unintended pregnancy could better foster family connectedness and decision-making in the family. Whtaker et al. (25) reported that young people are more open to discussion about SRH if they perceive the adult to be skilled, and open.

ACKNOWLEDGMENTS

To my supervisor, assistant professor Olanrewaju for your time and patience during the course of this research. I also wish to express my sincere thanks to the Babcock University for accepting me into the graduate program and for creating the platform for academic excellence. I am grateful to all the schools involved in this study for their maximum cooperation and support given to me along the way. A very special gratitude goes out to my parents for helping and providing the funding for the work. With a special mention to Chaplain Samuelle Ngo Ikouba Nfor and professor James Ogunji. The success of this research work cannot be emphasised without you two in the picture. A special thanks to my esteemed classmate, especially Ololade Ogunsami and Kukoyi Olasumbo. It was fantastic to have the opportunity to work with you. This study was self-sponsored. The authors declare that they have no conflict of interest. Informed consent was obtained from each individual participant involved in this study. This study was conducted in accordance with the 1964 Declaration of Helsinki and its subsequent amendments. No animal was involved in this study.

REFERENCES

[1] Adefioye OA, Arulogun OS. Attitudes towards mandatory pre-marital HIV testing among unmarried youths in Ibadan Northwest Local Government Area, Nigeria. Afr J Reprod Health 2010;14:83-94.

[2] United Nations Children's Fund (UNICEF) *Adolescents and young people – UNICEF data* 2017. URL: https://data.unicef.org/.

[3] Badru T, Mwaisaka J, Khamofu H, Agbakwuru C, Adedokun O, Pandey SR. et al. HIV comprehensive knowledge and prevalence among young adolescents in Nigeria: evidence from Akwa Ibom AIDS indicator survey, 2017. BMC Public Health 2020;45:20.

[4] Lynsey C. One-step forward, two steps back. Nine out of ten adolescent deaths due to AIDS are in Africa. Quartz Africa 2017. URL: https://qz.com/africa/1144158/hiv-aids-statistics-in-africa-nine-out-of-ten-adolescent-deaths-due-to-virus/.

[5] Slogrove AL, Mahy M, Armstrong A, Davies MA. Living and dying to be counted: What we know about the epidemiology of the global adolescent HIV epidemic. J Int AIDS Soc 2017;20:21520.

[6] UNAIDS. Federal Ministry of Health. New survey results indicate that Nigeria has an HIV prevalence of 1.4% Abuja/Geneva; 2019. URL: http://www.unaids.org/en/resources/presscentre/pressreleaseandstatementarchive/2019/march/20190314_nigeria.

[7] UNAIDS. Ending the AIDS epidemic for adolescents, with adolescents. Geneva. 2019. URL: http://www.unaids.org/en/ resources/documents/2016/ending-AIDS-epidemic-adolescents.

[8] Enejoh V, Pharr J, Mavegam BO, Olutola A, Karick H, Ezeanolue EE. Impact of self-esteem on risky sexual behaviors among Nigerian adolescents. AIDS Care 2016;28:672–6.

[9] Dauda RS, Olaniyan O. Macroeconomic impact of HIV/AIDS in Nigeria: error correction modeling (ECM) approach. Adv Soc Sci Res J *2017;4:*31-48.

[10] Dauda RS. Impact of HIV/AIDS epidemic on human capital development in West Africa. Int J Health Plann Manage *2018;*33*:*460-78.

[11] Federal Ministry of Health (FMOH). National HIV/AIDS and Reproductive Health Survey. Abuja, Nigeria. 2012. URL: https://www.unaids.org/sites/default/files/country/documents/NGA_narrative_report_2014.pdf

[12] Nigeria HIV/AIDS Indicator and Impact Survey (NAIIS). Preliminary findings, South West Zone - March 2018. URL: https://www.naiis.ng/resource/factsheet/NAIIS%20PA%20NATIONAL%20FACTSHEET%20FINAL.pdf.

[13] National AIDS/STDs Control Programme (NASCP). Federal Ministry of Health, Nigeria: National HIV/Syphilis Seroprevalence Sentinel Survey, process and findings 2008. URL: https://naca.gov.ng/ANC_2008_survey.pdf.

[14] Asefa A, Beyene H. Awareness and knowledge on timing of mother-to-child transmission of HIV among antenatal care attending women in Southern Ethiopia: a cross sectional study. Reprod Health 2013;10:66.

[15] Mwamwenda T. University Students' Knowledge of HIV/AIDS at an Adventist University in Tanzania. *Mediterr J Soc Sci* 2014;5:816.

[16] Olabode A, Olagoke MA. Urban-rural differentials in HIV/AIDS knowledge of Nigerian senior secondary school students. Int J Health Sci 2016;4:35-41.

[17] Haddison EC, Nguefack – Tsague G, Noubom M, Mbacham W, Ndumbe PM, Mbopi-Keou FX. Voluntary counseling and testing for HIV among high school students in Tiko health district, Cameroon. Pan Afr Med J 2012;13:18.

[18] Nubed CK, Akoachere JTK. Knowledge, attitudes and practices regarding HIV/AIDS among senior secondary school students in Fako Division, South West Region, Cameroon. BMC Public Health 2016;16:847.

[19] Adelakun K, Malachy NO. School location and secondary school students' awareness of human immunodeficiency virus/acquired immune deficiency syndrome (HIV/AIDS) in Imo State of Nigeria. J Educ Soc Res 2011;1:39-47.

[20] Bamise OF, Bamise CT, Adedigba MA. Knowledge of HIV/AIDS among secondary school adolescents in Osun state, Nigeria. Niger J Clin Pract 2011;14:338-44.

[21] Stonbraker S, Smaldone A, Luft H, Cushman LF, Nadal L, Halpern M, et al. Associations between health literacy, HIV-related knowledge, and information behavior among persons living with HIV in the Dominican Republic. Public Health Nurs 2018;35:166–75.

[22] Kirby DB, Laris BA, Rolleri LA. Sex and HIV education programs: their impact on sexual behaviors of young people throughout the world. J Adolesc Health 2007;40:206–17.

[23] Choy KK, Rene TJ, Khan SA. Beliefs and attitudes of medical students from public and private universities in Malaysia towards individuals with HIV/AIDS. ScientificWorldJournal 2013;2:462826.

[24] Wamoyi JW, Ferwick A, Urassa M, Zaba B, Stones W. Parent-child communication about sexual and reproductive health in rural Tanzania: Implications for young people's sexual health interventions. Reprod Health 2010;7:6.

[25] Whitaker DJ, Miller KS, Levin ML, Xu X. Patterns of condom use among adolescents: the impact of mother-adolescent communication. Am J Public Health 1988;88:1542-44.

In: Pediatrics and Adolescent Health ISBN: 978-1-68507-490-6
Editors: J. Merrick and M. Morad

Chapter 14

SELF-ESTEEM AND ASSERTIVENESS AS PREDICTORS OF INTENTIONS TO PRACTICE SAFE SEXUAL BEHAVIOR AMONG ADOLESCENTS IN SELECTED SECONDARY SCHOOLS IN IBADAN, OYO STATE

Catherine O Agbede, PhD
and Ololade O Ogunsanmi*, PhD
Department of Public Health, School of Public and Allied Health,
Babcock University, Nigeria

ABSTRACT

Adolescents are vulnerable to negative outcomes of sexual-risk behaviors because of their curiosity and impulsivity. The ability to communicate with one's sexual partner about condom use will build adolescents' intention to practice safe sexual behaviors (SSB). In this

* Corresponding Author's E-mail: ogunsanmio@babcock.edu.ng.

chapter we try to determine the relationship between self-esteem and assertiveness with intention to practice safe sexual behaviors. Study group: One hundred and forty-four in-school adolescents from public senior secondary schools in Ibadan, Oyo State, Nigeria. Methods: Design was descriptive cross-sectional, selecting four schools through a multi-stage sampling technique from four (4) semi-urban local government areas of the city. A validated instrument was used to collect data on sexual experience, self-esteem, assertiveness and intention to practice SSB. Frequencies, descriptive statistics, correlation and regression were conducted using the Statistical Package for Social Sciences (SPSS). Ethical considerations were ensured. Results: The mean±SD age of the adolescents was 15.94±1.57; 74 (51.4%) were males and 70 (48.6%), females. Self-esteem, assertiveness and intention to practice SSB which were measured on 30-point, 52-point and 24-point rating scales had mean±SD scores of 16.22±3.209, 29.97±7.653 and 15.98±3.709 respectively. Self-esteem had a significant relationship with the intention to practice SSB but only predicted 4.1% of the variation in intention to practice SSB ($r = 0.202$; $r^2 = 0.041$; $p = 0.015$). Gender and assertiveness did not predict the intention to practice SSB. Conclusions: The ability to communicate with one's sexual partner about condom use will build adolescents' intention to practice safe sexual behaviors.

INTRODUCTION

Adolescent sexuality continues to be an important topic which generates both public health and social concerns. This is attributable to its strong relationship with negative outcomes like adolescent pregnancy, truncated education and sexually transmitted infections (STI). Sexual-risk behaviors which include the number and types of relationships, early age at first sexual intercourse, unprotected sexual intercourse with 'at risk' sexual partners, inconsistent use of condom during sex, transactional sex engagement, unprotected anal sex and untreated STIs (1) are commonly practiced by adolescents.

Adolescence is a stage during which health habits which have a strong connection with future wellbeing are molded. The timing and nature of an adolescent's first sexual intercourse is a key variable which can predict high risk sexual behaviors. Sexual debut is one of life's significant events and it serves as a foundation for the subsequent pattern of sexual behavior among adolescents (2). A considerable proportion of young people in Nigeria is sexually active and increasingly engage in risky sexual behaviors (3-5). Adolescents are particularly vulnerable to sexually transmitted infections (STIs) because of their curiosity and impulsivity hence, the increase in the prevalence of human immunodeficiency syndrome (HIV) yearly (6). The high rate of new HIV infections and fertility among adolescents in the Sub-Saharan African region (7) has influenced a need to address these sexual and reproductive health challenges experienced by adolescents. Nearly 90% of adolescents living with HIV infections live in Sub-Saharan Africa; about 11% of new HIV infections are among adolescents and adolescents in Nigeria account for 7% of the new HIV infections (8).

About 6% of teenagers in southwest of Nigeria have begun childbearing and specifically, Oyo State has the third highest rate of teenage mothers with rate of 8.2% (9). Young people in the rural residences have a 52.3% rate of unmet need for contraceptives while their counterparts in the urban areas recorded a rate of 45.7% (9). Pregnancy has become a global problem among teenagers; it has eaten deep into the annals of most secondary schools in Nigeria. In Oyo State generally, it is observed that many teenage girls in the secondary school have dropped out due to early pregnancy. Adolescents who initiate sex at younger ages may be at increased risk for unintended pregnancy because they are less likely to practice effective contraception.

Understanding psychosocial theories and their applications have helped to highlight some of the individual and social factors which influence sexual behaviors. Internalized and psychosocial traits including a set of sexual self-perceptions, such as sexual self-esteem, sexual self-efficacy, sexual assertiveness and sexual self-beliefs, have been shown to have close relationship with individual sexual behaviors among adolescents (10). Low levels of sexual self-perceptions may make adolescents vulnerable to the aforementioned risky sexual behaviors.

Generally, self-esteem is described as the evaluation of oneself; how one feels about his/herself in almost any situation. High self-esteem is manifested by acceptance of responsibility for one's own actions, self-motivation, willingness to take reasonable risk, and taking command and control of one's personal life including health behaviors. Adolescents who have low self-esteem scores are more likely to be sexually active with higher sexual-risk behavior scores (11). These finding are consistent with other studies of self-esteem and RSB in adolescents (12, 13). A likely explanation for these findings is that adolescents with low self-esteem typically focus on trying to prove themselves or impress others. They generally lack confidence in themselves, often have doubts about their worth and thus more susceptible to pressure to engage in risky sex.

Sexual self-assertiveness is a sub-type of sexual communication which has been defined as a person's ability to communicate sexual needs and initiate sexual behavior with a partner. Sexual assertiveness is linked to one's insistence to engage in safe sex behaviors with a partner (14). Assertiveness also involves direct attempts to change partner's behavior if it conflicts with one's beliefs or attitudes. In the context of this study, sexual assertiveness will be the adolescents' ability to insist on practicing safe sexual intercourse, commitment to employ appropriate contraception, ability to initiate sex with a partner, ability to refuse unwanted sex, the capacity to communicate sexual desires, discuss sexual history and insist on one's right to practice safe sex.

It is imperative to pay crucial attention to the psychosocial factors (self-esteem, sexual assertiveness) that influence intentions to practice safe sex among adolescents in Nigeria. The purpose of the current study was to enhance the standing research on psychosocial factors' role in sexual behavior of adolescents by exploring the degree to which self-esteem and self-assertiveness influence the intention to practice safe sex among a sample of adolescents in Ibadan, Oyo State. In the present study, the psychosocial factors which are the independent variables of interest are self-esteem and self-assertiveness while the dependent variable was intention to practice safe sex behaviors. The dependent variables referred to the condom use intention, sexual partner limitations and sexual debut delay for non-sexually active adolescents. In line with the above discussions, we hypothesized that the adolescents' intention to engage in safe sexual practice will be positively and significantly predicted by the level of self-esteem. Secondly, the intention to practice safe will predicted by the level of assertiveness of the adolescents. Thirdly, sexually active adolescents' intention to practice safe sex will not be different from the non-sexually active.

OUR STUDY

Data was collected from in-school adolescents between in December, 2019. The study employed a descriptive cross-sectional survey design of adolescents studying in public senior secondary schools in Ibadan, Nigeria. Ibadan is the capital city of Oyo State with 5 urban local government areas and 6 semi urban respectively. Four schools were selected through a multi-stage sampling technique from four (4) semi-urban local government areas of the city. The adolescents were in the senior classes and within the age range of 10 and 19 years old which is the globally recognized age range for adolescents. Adolescents' participation was totally voluntary and the data used for the research was collected with a validated (Cronbach Alpha score = 0.73), self-administered and semi-structured instrument. The instrument solicited information on the adolescents' sexual experiences, self-esteem, sexual assertiveness and intention to practice safe sexual behaviors. Permission and consent for the study was obtained from the State Ministry of Health Ethics and Research Committee.

MEASURES

Sexual self-esteem was measured with the Rosenberg Self-Esteem Likert Scale comprising in total ten item statements which enquired on whether the individual strongly agreed, agreed, disagreed or strongly disagreed with the statements that enquired on their evaluations of themselves. The scale has an internal consistency score of 0.77 to 0.88. In scoring the items, the positive statements were given points as follows; Strongly Agree (SA) = 3, Agree (A) = 2, Disagree (D) = 1 and Strongly Disagree (SD) = 0 while the negative statements (items 18, 21, 22, 24 and 25) were reversed scored as follows; SA = 0, A = 1, D = 2 and SD = 3 and finally summing the numbers to get the score for the overall self-esteem. The scores were interpreted to mean that the higher the sum number, the higher the individual's self-esteem. A maximum score of 30 is expected for the self-esteem scale.

Sexual assertiveness was measured by adopting the Hulbert Index of Sexual Assertiveness (HISA). The HISA is comprised of 25 Likert-type questions with a published Cronbach's alpha of 0.92. The adolescents are to indicate their level of assertiveness by responding to the items using All of the time = AT; Most of the time = MT; Some of the time = ST; Rarely = R; Never = N. Twelve of the items are negatively constructed and the final scores will be computed on a scale of 100-points rating.

Seven items adapted from previous research and literature assessed participants' intentions to practice safe sexual behaviors in the future (i.e., over the coming six months). The section was grouped into the "condom use intention," "sexual intercourse delay" and "limit sexual partners." Sample items included "I will not have sex now because I want to wait until I am older," and "I will not have sex unless I use a condom." Scale responses were scored such that higher scores indicated more favorable intentions towards condom use over the next three months. In scoring the items, the positive statements were given points as follows; Strongly Agree (SA) = 3, Agree (A) = 2, Disagree (D) = 1 and Strongly Disagree (SD) = 0 while the negative statements (items 18, 21, 22, 24 and 25) were reversed scored as follows; SA = 0, A = 1, D = 2 and SD = 3.

Data analysis

The data were analyzed using the Statistical Package for Social Sciences (SPSS - version 22). Frequency counts was used in presenting results of the social demographic variables and sexual experience. The relationship between the continuous variables was measured with correlation and regression. Analysis of Variance (ANOVA) measured the relationship between the categorical and continuous variables.

Table 1. Demographic attributes of the adolescents

S/N	Variables	Frequency (N)	Percentage (%)
1	Gender		
	Male	74	51.4
	Female	70	48.6
2	Age		
	10 – 14	21	14.6
	15 – 19	123	85.4
3	Mean±SD Age	15.94±1.570	
4	Class		
	SS 1	44	30.6
	SS 2	48	33.3
	SS 3	52	36.1
5	Religion		
	Christianity	67	46.5
	Islam	74	51.4
	Traditional	3	2.1

FINDINGS

The descriptive analysis as presented in Table 1 showed that the mean±SD age of the adolescents was 15.94±1.570 with 51.4% being females and 48.6%, males. The students were distributed across the three (3) senior secondary school classes 1 (30.6), 2 (33.3) and 3 (36.1) with almost half of them (46.5%) reporting to be affiliated with the Christianity religion. We assessed the adolescents' sexual experience to have picture of the level of sexual exposure. Majority (84%) reported that they had never had a sexual intercourse. Among adolescents who had experienced a sexual intercourse, the mean±SD age at first sexual intercourse was 13.91±1.929 years. The results showed that among the adolescents who had had sex, money/gifts were the most common reason for the first sexual intercourse followed by peer pressure and rape (see Table 2). The proportion of adolescents who have had sex in the past 6 months before the study was 11.1% and 17.39% of the sexually experienced (n = 23) reported to have had sexual intercourse with someone older (5 years or more). Regarding the use of condoms during sexual intercourse, 34.78% of the sexually experienced (n = 23) adolescents reported to always use a condom while 65.22% stated otherwise. At last intercourse, 52.17% reported to have used a condom while 47.83% did not (see Table 2).

The responses to the items to measure the self-esteem of the adolescents were computed on a with the descriptive statistics presented in Table 3. The mean±SD values for self-esteem (16.22±3.209) and assertiveness (29.97±7.653) were low while the adolescents recorded a fairly good level of intention to practice safe sexual intercourse. Self-esteem had a positive significant relationship with the intention to use condom and the accumulated intention to practice safe sexual intercourse ($r = 0.202$; $p = 0.015$). Assertiveness had a positive significant relationship with the intention to delay sexual debut only. Gender also had no relationship with the intention to practice safe sexual behaviors ($F = 6.87$; $p = 0.409$). Further regression analysis was conducted to determine the level of variance in intention to practice safe sex caused by the level of self-esteem. Results showed that though there was a significant relationship between the variables; self-esteem predicted only 4.1% of the observed variation in the adolescents' intention to practice safe sex (r2 = 0.041; p-value = 0.015). While comparing the sexually active adolescents' intention to practice safer sexual behaviors and the non-sexually active students, it was observed that those for those had had a sexual intercourse, self-esteem contributes to 22.5% (R2 = 0.225) of the change that may be observed in their intention to practice safe sexual behaviors. For the adolescents who had never had a sexual intercourse, self-esteem predicted only 12.6% of their intentions (see Table 5).

Table 2. Responses to the sexual experience of the adolescents

S/N	ITEMS	Frequency (N)	Percentage (%)
1	Have you ever had sexual intercourse?		
	Yes	23	16.0
	No	121	84.0
2	Age at first sexual intercourse	Mean±SD = 13.91±1.929	
	Reason for first sexual intercourse		
	Never had sexual intercourse	121	84.0
	Peer pressure	6	4.2
	Curiosity	3	2.1
	Money/Gifts	9	6.3
	Personal Gain	1	0.7
	Rape	4	2.8
3	Have you had sexual intercourse in the past 6 months?		
	Yes	16	11.1
	No	128	88.9
4	How many sexual partners have you had in the past 6 months?		
	0	128	88.9
	1 - 5	16	11.1
	6 - 10	0	0.0
		N = 23	
5	Did you ever have sex with someone much older than you (5 years and above) in the past 6 months?		
	Yes	4	17.39
	No	19	82.61
6	Have you ever had unprotected sexual intercourse because you were intoxicated (drink or drugs)?		
	Yes	2	8.70
	No	21	91.30
7	Do you always use a condom during sexual intercourse?		
	Yes	8	34.78
	No	15	65.22
8	The last time you had sexual intercourse, did you or your partner use a condom?		
	Yes	12	52.17
	No	11	47.83

Table 3. Descriptive statistics of variables

Variables	Rating Scale	Mean	SD
Self Esteem	30 points	16.22	3.209
Assertiveness	52 points	29.97	7.653
Intention to Practice Safe Sex	24 points	15.98	3.709
Intention to Use Condoms	6 points	3.65	2.019
Intention to Delay Sexual Debut	15 points	10.63	3.045
Intention to Limit Sexual Partners	3 points	1.70	1.116

Table 4. Correlation between the dependent and independent variables

	Intention to Use Condom	Intention to Limit Partners	Intention to Delay Sexual Debut	Intention to Practice Safe Sex
Self-esteem				
Pearson	0.278	-0.065	0.086	0.202
p-value	0.01*	0.437	0.306	0.015*
Assertiveness				
Pearson	-0.056	-0.020	0.171	0.004
p-value	0.506	0.810	0.041*	0.958
Gender				
F value	6.684	5.522	1.064	6.87
p-value	0.011*	0.020*	0.304	0.409

* Sig at $p<0.05$.

Obtained by Pearson Correlation.

Table 5. Regression analysis between self-esteem and intention to practice safe sex

	df	R	R Square	F	p-value
Intention to Practice Safe Sex/Self-esteem					
Sexually Active (N = 23)	22	0.474	0.225	6.081	0.000
Non-Sexually Active (N = 121)	120	0.354	0.126	17.094	0.000
Total (144)	144	0.202	0.041	6.035	0.000

* Sig at $p<0.05$.

Obtained by Regression.

DISCUSSION

This study investigated the practices of safe sexual behaviors among adolescents and the psychosocial factors that predict intension to practice safe sexual behaviors. The participants were recruited from four semi-urban local government areas across the city, Ibadan. The adolescents were currently enrolled in secondary schools during the period were in senior classes. The mean±SD age of the adolescents was 15.94±1.570 years which was similar to the mean age of adolescents reported in several studies (15-17). The similarity in age group is due to the fact that most adolescents in secondary schools, especially senior classes in their mid-adolescence age and complete the secondary school education by late adolescence.

The study revealed that a total of 23 (19.17%) of the adolescents had engaged in a sexual intercourse and the mean±SD age at sexual debut was 13.91±1.929. This finding is similar to the mean ages reported in Ekiti State (15), also in the southwestern region of the country. In a country representative study, Yaya and Bishwajit, (18) reported that adolescents, particularly girls were experiencing sexual debut before reaching 15 years. In a community-based study conducted to determine the age at sexual debut of the residents, it was reported that the mean age was 17 years.

Correlation analysis showed that only self-esteem had a relationship with intention to practice safe sexual behaviors. The findings of this study indicate that self-esteem could only predict 4.1% of the change in intention. This is a low correlational value and it suggests that there are other factors which may influence the adolescents' intention to practice safe sexual behaviors. Other researches regarding self-esteem and RSB in adolescences has found a positive relationship between high self-esteem and lower RSB (13, 19). Specifically, some researches some findings have supported the relationship between lower self-esteem, earlier sex initiation, history of risky sexual partners and unprotected intercourse (13). Adolescents who have a low self-esteem may also be predisposed to unintended pregnancies because of their lack of confidence in themselves inability to expresses a want for or negotiate condom use. Sexual initiation at a young age is markedly correlated with high chances of the individuals having longer exposure to the negative outcomes of high-risk sexual behaviors and more pregnancies. Also, an earlier study found an association between lower self-esteem and high risk for pregnancy in late adolescence and early adulthood (20).

Lower self-esteem in a family setting and among peers influences low levels of self-worth which is a component of self-perception. A study conducted by Enejoh et al. (11) revealed that adolescents with low self-esteem were more likely to be sexually active and to have higher mean RSB score. These finding are consistent with other studies of self-esteem and RSB in adolescents (12, 13). A likely explanation for these findings is that adolescents with low self-esteem typically focus on trying to prove themselves or impress others. They generally lack confidence in themselves, often have doubts about their worth and thus more susceptible to pressure to engage in risky sex.

The ability to communicate with one's sexual partner about condom use will build adolescents' intention to practice safe sexual behaviors. The behavioral skills developed by adolescents highlights the ability to be assertive in one's communications to a partner about the intention to use a condom and the ability to negotiate condom use in the face of dissatisfaction or objection from the partner. Sexual communication has evolved from asking partners about their sexual history to expressing desires and being assertive. Being assertive, as a behavioral component does not only translate to personal beliefs or confidence. Also, the ability to communicate effectively with one's partner, engage in actual preventive behaviors such as condom use is the goal of the research. Adolescents may be unaware of their risks or underestimate their vulnerability; it is thus imperative that sexually active individuals develop communication skills which can enable them to request that a partner for condom use, and to negotiate condom use in the face of partner dissatisfaction.

This study was conducted to generate vital evidence on the relationship between adolescents' sexual behaviors and their self-esteem and assertiveness and several limitations need to be acknowledged. Due to the design of the study, the findings cannot be generalized to other locations of the country, Nigeria. The existence of response bias could also have affected the administration of the instrument for data collection. The responses on the sexual behaviors is based solely on information reported by the adolescents and may have meaning influenced by socially accepted values.

Conclusion

Based on the findings of the study, it can be said that self-esteem significantly influences the intentions of adolescents to practice safe sexual behaviors. It was also revealed that sexual assertiveness had no relationship with the intention of adolescents to practice safe sexual behaviors. High self-esteem should be regarded as a protective factor in the field of sexual and reproductive health. These will promote health sexual behaviors which typically aim to delay sexual debut and increase condom use. For adolescents who may be sexually active, developing a protective psychological skill will help them in making informed choices and be able to negotiate sexual activities with their partners. Subsequently, interventions aimed at promotion of positive and high self-esteem are imperative among adolescents.

Acknowledgments

We would like to express our gratitude to the Oyo State Ministry of Education for the permission granted to conduct the study, teachers and students of the selected secondary schools. We are grateful to the research assistants for assisting us in the data collection and data entry.

This study was independently funded by the researchers. The authors declare that they have no conflict of interest. Informed consent was obtained from each individual who participated in this study and conducted in accordance with the 1964 Declaration of Helsinki and its subsequent amendments.

REFERENCES

[1] Abdulai MA, Baiden F, Afari-Asiedu S, Gyabaa-Febir L, Adjei KK, Mahama E, et al. The risk of sexually transmitted infection and its influence on condom use among pregnant women in the Kintampo north municipality of Ghana. J Sex Transm Dis 2017;2017:8642685.

[2] Wight D, Parkes A, Strange V, Allen E, Bonell C, Henderson M. The quality of young people's heterosexual relationships: A longitudinal analysis of characteristics shaping subjective experience. Perspect Sex Reprod Health 2008;40:226–37.

[3] Okereke C. assessing the prevalence and determinants of adolescents' unintended pregnancy and induced abortion in Owerri, Nigeria. J Biosoc Sci Suppl 2010;42(5):619-32.

[4] Cherie A, Berhane Y. Knowledge of sexually transmitted infections and barriers to seeking health services among high school adolescents in Addis Ababa, Ethiopia. J AIDS Clin Res 2012;3:153.

[5] Ajide KB, Balogun FM. Knowledge of HIV and intention to engage in risky sexual behavior and practices among senior school adolescents in Ibadan, Nigeria. Arch Basic Appl Med 2018;6(1);3–8.

[6] Barnabas SI, Dabee S, Passmore JAS, Jaspan HB, Lewis DA, Jaumdally SZ et al. Converging epidemics of sexually transmitted infections and bacterial vaginosis in southern African female adolescents at risk of HIV. Int J STD AIDS 2018;29(6):531–9.

[7] UNAIDS. Prevention gap report: UNAIDS; 2016. URL: http://www.unaids.org/sites/default/files/mediaasset/2016-prevention-gap-report_en.pdf.

[8] UNICEF. Adolescent HIV Prevention, July 2019. URL: https://data.unicef.org/topic/hivaids/adolescents-young-people/#status.

[9] National Population Commission (NPC) [Nigeria] and ICF. Nigeria Demographic and Health Survey, 2018.

[10] Bui TC, Markham CM, Ross MW, Williams ML, Beasley R.P, Tran LT, et al. Perceived gender inequality, sexual communication self-efficacy, and sexual

behavior among female undergraduate students in the Mekong Delta of Vietnam. Sex Health 2012;9:314-22

[11] Enejoh V, Pharr J, Mavegam BO, Olutola A, Karick H, Ezeanolue EE. Impact of self-esteem on risky sexual behaviors among Nigerian adolescents. AIDS Care 2016;28(5):672–76.

[12] Sangowawa AO, Adebiyi AO. Factors associated with sexual abstinence among out-of-school females in a transitional town in Oyo state, south-western Nigeria. Health Care Women Int 2013;34(10):917–32.

[13] Ethier KA, Kershaw TS, Lewis JB, Milan S, Niccolai LM, Ickovics JR. Self-esteem, emotional distress and sexual behavior among adolescent females: Interrelationships and temporal effects. J Adolesc Health 2006;38(3):268–74.

[14] Widman L, Noar SM, Choukas-Bradley S, Francis DB. Adolescent sexual health communication and condom use: A meta-analysis. Health Psychol 2014;33:1113-24.

[15] Durowade KA, Babatunde OA, Omokanye LO, Elegbede OE, Ayodele LM, Adewoye KR, et al. Early sexual debut: prevalence and risk factors among secondary school students in Ido-ekiti, Ekiti state, South-West Nigeria. Afr Health Sci 2017;17(3):614-22.

[16] Chilisa R., Tlhabano K, Vista C, Pheko M, Losike N, Mosime S, et al. Self-efficacy, self-esteem and the intention to practice safe sex among Batswana adolescents. Int J Humanit Soc Sci 2014;9(2):87-95.

[17] Espada J, Morales A, Guillén-Riquelme A, Ballester-Arnal R, Orgilés M. Predicting condom use in adolescents: A test of three socio-cognitive models using a structural equation modeling approach. BMC Public Health 2016;16:35.

[18] Yaya S, Bishwajit G. Age at first sexual intercourse and multiple sexual partnerships among women in Nigeria: a cross-sectional analysis. Front Med 2018;5:171.

[19] Sánchez MTR, Alvarez IT, Sánchez MPB, Casal GB. Social support, self-esteem and depression: Relationship with risk for sexually transmitted infections/ HIV transmission. Int J Clin Health Psychol 2013;13(3):181–8.

[20] Boden JM, Horwood LJ. Self-esteem, risky sexual behavior, and pregnancy in a New Zealand birth cohort. Arch Sex Behav 2006;35(5):549-60.

In: Pediatrics and Adolescent Health ISBN: 978-1-68507-490-6
Editors: J. Merrick and M. Morad

Chapter 15

EFFECT OF NUTRITION EDUCATION AND MOBILE TEXT MESSAGES ON UNDERGRADUATES' EATING PRACTICES AND PERCEPTION OF RISK IN OYO STATE, NIGERIA

Olasumbo Bilikisu Kukoyi *
and Ademola Mufutau Amosu, PhD
Department of Public Health, School of Public and Allied Health,
Babcock University, Nigeria

* Corresponding Author's E-mail: kukoyiolasumbo@gmail.com.

ABSTRACT

Young adults in the university are vulnerable in their eating habits for various reasons which include their deficiency in knowledge about what constitute healthy food that could influence their eating habits and their perception of risk by unhealthy dietary choices. The broad objective for this study was to evaluate the effect of nutrition education and mobile text messages on undergraduates eating practices and perception of risk in Oyo state, Nigeria. The study used a quasi-experimental design, comprising of three experimental groups and one control group. The study population were undergraduates in selected universities in Oyo state. This study was implemented in three phases: Baseline survey/data collection, intervention/evaluation and follow-up evaluation. A quantitative data collection instrument was used for data collection. The data obtained from completed questionnaires was collated and analysed using Statistical Package for Social Science (SPSS) version 23.0. There were 100 respondents recruited for this study with a mean age of 19.80 ± 2.22 years, however, there were 94 respondents at the follow-up stage of the study, indicating a 6% loss to follow-up. Respondents perception and eating practice was poor at baseline. However, eating practice and perception of risk significantly increased across the experimental groups at follow-up. Combination of both nutrition education and mobile text messages improved respondents' eating practice and perception of risk more than isolation of nutrition education and mobile phone communication interventions separately.

INTRODUCTION

Young adults in the university setting are vulnerable in their eating habits for various reasons which include their deficiency in knowledge about what constitute healthy food that could influence their eating habits. Financial aspects might also play a role, as fats and sweets cost less, whereas many healthier foods cost more and students also face academic responsibilities that may generate stress and lead to changes in eating habits (1). In addition, students' eating behaviour could be affected by university characteristics such as students' societies, university lifestyle and exams and by the institution nutrition environment and its contribution to adoption of healthy/unhealthy eating habits (2).

The dangers associated with unhealthy eating practices supersedes that of overweight and obesity, but also psychosocial-related health problems, which include body image dissatisfaction, suicide and can affect perceptions of body weight and the influence of body image on self-esteem, happiness and wellbeing (3). Immediate health problems, such as reduced capacity for learning and work, to a growing burden of modifiable non-communicable diseases (NCDs) can also occur.

In the past three decades, global overweight (body mass index (BMI) $\geq$25 kg/m^2) increased from 28.8% to 36.9% in males and from 29.8% to 38.0% in females, while age-standardized obesity (BMI $\geq$30 kg/m^2) increased from 3.2% to 10.8% in males and from 6.4% to 14.9% in females. This is attributed to the rapid shift in dietary patterns currently adopted by many parts of sub-Saharan Africa, where people have gone from consuming traditional diets high in cereals, fibre, fruits and vegetables to a more Western diet consisting of foods high in sugar, saturated fat, salt, and animal proteins but low in fruits, vegetables, and other plant-based foods, resulting in low dietary fibre, non-starchy polysaccharides, and resistant starch. This change in diet that occurs as countries develop is what is generally referred to as the nutrition transition (4).

To facilitate the adoption of healthy eating practice among young adults, nutrition education is essential, through which young adults will be intimated on what constitutes a healthy diet and the importance of diet on their growth and development, and also for supporting the development of healthful lifestyles, preventing weight-related problems, reducing disease risk and ensuring that all needs are met for growth and development (5).

The dietary practices of young adults in Nigeria is undergoing a rapid shift to less-healthy diets (consisting of processed foods, fast food, and increase intake of sugar-sweetened beverages). These group of people are at the centre of diet related non-communicable diseases which has taken over communicable diseases as the leading causes of morbidity and mortality in Nigeria. According to the Global Status Report on Non-communicable diseases, Nigeria had an estimated 792,600 NCDs related deaths in 2008 and this high mortality figure is linked to four modifiable risk factors namely *physical inactivity, unhealthy diets, tobacco and harmful alcohol use*. These risk factors are said to be initiated during adolescence and set the stage for unhealthy behaviours which persist into adulthood and diseases later in life (6). The broad objective for the study was to evaluate the effect of nutrition education and mobile text messages on undergraduates eating practices and perception of risk in Oyo state, Nigeria.

OUR STUDY

This study used a quasi-experimental design (quantitative method), comprising of three experimental groups and one control group (experimental group 1: Nutrition education and mobile text messages (NE & MTM); experimental group 2: Nutrition education alone (NE alone); experimental group 3: Mobile text messages alone (MTM alone). The study population were undergraduates in selected universities in Oyo state. There are nine universities in the state (two public and seven private). The inclusion criteria for participants in this study were as follows:

1. The students must be fully registered undergraduate students of the selected tertiary institutions and owns a mobile phone
2. The students must be within the age bracket of young adulthood (16-30 years) and be interested in healthy eating practices.

There was no given estimate of the prevalence of the eating practice of university students in Oyo-state, thus, the sample size was determined using Power formula for computation of sample size. This sample size is just for one population (one university), therefore the total size was multiplied by four to get the total sample size for all the targeted population in the four selected universities.

$$n = \frac{(Z_\alpha + Z_\beta)^2 \times P_0(1 - P_0)}{(P_1 - P_0)^2}$$

Z_α = 95% confidence interval i.e., 1.96

Z_β = 80% i.e., 0.84 (Power to detect changes in the outcome variable and avoid type II error)

P_0 = prevalence (at 50%)

P_1 = 80% (desired level of outcome variable i.e., adherence to healthy eating practices)

$$n = \frac{(1.96 + 0.84)^2 \times 0.5(1 - 0.5)}{(0.8 - 0.5)^2}$$

$$\frac{(2.8)^2 \times 0.5(0.5)}{(0.8 - 0.5)^2}$$

$$\frac{7.84 \times 0.25}{0.09}$$

$$=21.78 \simeq 22$$

The minimum sample size is 22. 10% of the minimum sample size was added to take care of attrition. The total number of participants after adding 10% of 22 was = 22 + 2.2 ≃ 25. Based on this computation a total number of 100 participants (25 X 4) from the four universities was enrolled for this study (representing 25 people per group)

Sampling technique

A list of universities in Oyo state was obtained from the state ministry of education, science and technology. First, stratified sampling technique was use to select the two government and two private universities for this study in Oyo state. By simple random sampling technique using the balloting method among the nine schools given, Ajayi Crowther University, University of Ibadan, Lead City University and Ladoke Akintola University of Technology was selected. Secondly, the selected universities were then randomly assigned to either experimental or control group.

Selection of respondents

Postal advertisement and flyers was circulated around the schools selected to recruit respondents for this study. Interested participants were screened to know if they are eligible for the study. In order to make sure that both gender is fully represented in the study, the participant was selected by means of non-probability method using convenience sampling technique. In each group the first 12 males or 13 females that meets the inclusion criteria were recruited for this study and vice versa. The advertisement contained the following information: The name and address of the researcher; A summary of purpose of the research; Basic eligibility criteria; The benefit of participating in the research; The time or other commitment required of the participant; and the name and phone number of the person to contact for further information.

This study was implemented in three phases: Baseline survey/data collection, intervention/evaluationand follow-up evaluation. A quantitative data collection instrument was used for data collection. Instrument was developed using information gathered from review of literature. The instrument was sectioned as follows:

- Section A: Socio-demographic characteristics of the participants that are relevant to the study which included the age, gender, marital status, religion, ethnicity and more.
- Section B: Perception of risk to life by unhealthy dietary choices which was operationalized by sub-variables of perceived susceptibility of the effect of unhealthy eating practices on health; perceived severity/seriousness of the effect of unhealthy eating practices on health; perceived benefits of eating healthy; and perceived barriers towards healthy eating practices. The sub domains had six (susceptibility, severity, benefit) and seven

(barrier) Likert questions respectively operationalizing them, translating to 18 and 21-points rating scale respectively. Therefore, together this variable will consist of 25 Likert questions measured on a 75-point rating scale of strongly agree (SA), agree (A), disagree (D) and strongly disagree (SD). The scale was represented as strongly agree (SA) as 1, agree (A) as 2, disagree (D) as 3 and strongly disagree (SD) as 4.

- Section C: Self-reported eating practices. This was operationalized in the section H of the instrument that asked questions about their behaviour regarding healthy diet measured on a 54 points rating scale. This variable was measured using an 18-Likert questions of never (N), rarely (R), often (O), and always (A). The scale was represented as never (N) as 1, rarely (R) as 2, often (O) as 3, and always (A) as 4.

To ascertain the reliability of the instrument, a pilot-test was first conducted for internal consistency of the instrument using 10% of the total projected sample size (10 undergraduate students) from Olabisi Onabanjo University Ogun-state. Thereafter, a test re-test was conducted for reliability of the instrument also using 10% of the anticipated sample size (10 undergraduate students) from Olabisi Onabanjo University Ogun-state. It was ensured that the sample for both the pilot-test and test-retest had the same characteristics as the study population.

The data from the test-retest was statistically analysed using Cronbach alpha standard score to test its reliability. After necessary adjustment, the Cronbach values were found to be between 0.70 and 0.81 for all the constructs in the questionnaire which shows good fit of the instrument. This study obtained ethical approval from Babcock University Health Research and Ethics Committee (BUHREC) with reference number BUHREC492/19 and Oyo State Ethics Review Committee under the Ministry of Health, Department of Planning, Research and Statistics Division with reference number AD/13/479/1486. Permission to conduct the study was also obtained from the dean of students' affairs in the various universities used for this study. All persons used for this study were informed that their participation is voluntary and inform consent was sought from all participants prior to their participation. Confidentiality of participants were maintained as no personal identifying information was collected on the questionnaire. Special care was taken to ensure that there was no false compensation or inducement as a means of recruitment or as a way of keeping the study respondents in the study.

Data collection procedure

The selected schools were visited earlier to get information and also seek permission from the relevant authorities for easy data collection. The instrument designed for the study was used to collect data. It was done at three points during the study; the baseline, immediate post-intervention and at 8th week follow up. Four research assistants (undergraduates) were recruited for this study.

Content of the training manual for the class room instruction intervention

- Module I: (i) Why nutrition matters (ii) The relationship between diet and health (iii) The food guide pyramid
- Module II: (i) Nutrients and their food sources (ii) Meaning of healthy balanced diet (iii) Diet diversity
- Module III: (i) Healthy dietary practices (ii) Meaning and component of healthy eating (iii) Importance of breakfast, lunch and dinner
- Module IV: (i) Relationship between disease and nutrition (ii) Detrimental effects of sugary foods and drinks (iii) hazards of fast food

- Module V: (i) Finding and choosing healthy foods (ii) Daily dietary needs for young adults (iii) Body image dissatisfaction
- Module VI: (i) Importance of fruits and vegetables and improving fruits and vegetables consumption (ii) barriers to fruits and vegetables consumption (iii) Meaning of food safety (iv) Hygiene practices during meal preparation and safeguarding of food.

Content of text messages

The healthy eating tips text messages (GO NOURISH) was based on packages from the classroom instructions (messages on healthy choices when eating out, the food guide pyramid, nutritional needs of young adults, hazards of fast food, and hygiene practices during preparation and safeguarding of food) was prepared and edited before final dissemination.

The text messages were sent using the bulk SMS platform and was sent every Monday, Wednesday and Friday between 4-6 am to ensure that the participant will adhere to good nutrition before eating during the day. The calculation was for them to wake up in the morning to read their healthy eating messages before commencing the day's activities in order for them to make good nutrition choices.

Data analysis

The data obtained from completed questionnaires was collated and analysed using Statistical Package for Social Science (SPSS) version 23.0. Data that was entered were subjected to descriptive (i.e., frequency, percentage, means, standard deviation, standard error) and inferential (i.e., t-test, ANOVA) statistical analyses at $p \leq 0.05$.

FINDINGS

There were 100 respondents recruited for this study with a mean age of 19.80 ± 2.22 years, however, there were 94 respondents at the follow up stage of the study, indicating a 6% loss to follow-up. Across both levels, majority of the respondents were of Christian religious belief (baseline: 85%; endline: 81.9%). All participants in this study were single at baseline and endline (100%) while undergraduates in the 100 level of education were the major participants in this study at baseline and endline (32% and 29.8% respectively) (see Table 1).

Table 1. Socio-demographic characteristics of respondents

Demographics Characteristics	Baseline		Endline	
	No.	%	No.	%
Age*				
Less than 19 years	52	52.0	35	37.2
19 years and above	48	48.0	59	62.8
Sex				
Female	66	66.0	45	47.9
Male	34	34.0	49	52.1
Marital status				
Single	100	100.0	94	100
Religion				
Christianity	85	85.0	77	81.9
Islam	15	15.0	14	14.9
Academic level				
100 level	32	32.0	28	29.8
200 level	20	20.0	24	25.5
300 level	15	15.0	20	21.3
400 level	29	29.0	19	20.2
500 level	4	4.0	3	3.2
Ethnicity				
Yoruba	65	65.0	60	63.8
Igbo	12	12.0	19	20.2
Hausa	4	4.0	1	1.1
Others	19	19.0	14	14.9
Residency				
Hostel	88	88.0	84	89.4
Town	12	12.0	10	10.6

Perception at baseline

Table 2 illustrates respondents' perception. Assessing the respondents' perceived susceptibility to the effect of unhealthy eating practices on their health, it was found that while a higher proportion (44%) of the respondents in the control group strongly agreed that it is impossible they fall sick as a result of diabetes despite high consumption of sugar, fewer respondents strongly agreed in the NE&MTM and MTM alone group at 20% and 24% respectively. Furthermore, a higher proportion of respondents in the control, NE alone and MTM alone groups at 44%, 40% and 40% respectively disagreed to being worried that their unhealthy eating practices can lead to being obese.

Table 2. Respondents' level of perception at baseline

Variables	NE & MTM		NE alone		MTM alone		Control	
	No.	%	No.	%	No.	%	No.	%
Perceived susceptibility								
In my family we eat alot of sugar and nothing happens to us, so it's impossible I fall sick as a result of diabetes	5	20.0	12	48.0	6	24.0	11	44.0
Strongly Agree	2	8.0	2	8.0	1	4.0	1	4.0
Agree	8	32.0	9	36.0	10	40.0	11	44.0
Disagree	10	40.0	2	8.0	8	32.0	2	4.0
Strongly disagree								
Am worried that my unhealthy eating practices can lead to me being obese								
Strongly Agree	5	20.0	3	12.0	4	16.0	2	8.0
Agree	11	44.0	4	16.0	8	32.0	8	32.0
Disagree	2	8.0	10	40.0	10	40.0	11	44.0
Strongly disagree	7	28.0	8	32.0	3	12.0	4	16.0
Perceived Severity								
I think there is nothing wrong in eating lots of salt and sugar								
Strongly Agree	2	8.0	2	8.0	8	32.0	6	24.0
Agree	4	16.0	3	12.0	7	28.0	6	24.0
Disagree	8	32.0	14	56.0	7	28.0	10	40.0
Strongly disagree	11	44.0	6	24.0	3	12.0	3	12.0

Table 2. (Continued)

Variables	NE & MTM		NE alone		MTM alone		Control	
	No.	%	No.	%	No.	%	No.	%
I feel if I take soft drinks as often as possible, there will be no health consequences now or later in life								
Strongly Agree	5	20.0	8	32.0	10	40.0	8	32.0
Agree	3	12.0	3	12.0	3	12.0	6	24.0
Disagree	8	32.0	9	36.0	8	32.0	9	36.0
Strongly disagree	9	36.0	5	20.0	4	16.0	2	8.0
Perceived benefit								
I do not think that healthy food can prevent diseases								
Strongly Agree	3	12.0	0	0.0	0	0.0	3	12.0
Agree	6	24.0	8	32.0	6	24.0	8	32.0
Disagree	9	36.0	13	52.0	14	56.0	9	36.0
Strongly disagree	7	28.0	4	16.0	5	20.0	5	20.0
Consuming a healthy diet will help in lowering my cholesterol level								
Strongly Agree	3	12.0	2	8.0	0	0.0	4	16.0
Agree	11	44.0	1	4.0	3	12.0	6	24.0
Disagree	4	16.0	11	44.0	12	48.0	10	40.0
Strongly disagree	7	28.0	11	44.0	10	40.0	5	20.0
A healthy diet reduces my risk of developing cardiovascular disease								
Strongly Agree	1	4.0	0	0.0	1	4.0	0	0.0
Agree	14	56.0	11	44.0	14	56.0	14	56.0
Disagree	10	40.0	13	52.0	9	36.0	10	40.0
Strongly disagree	0	0.0	1	4.0	1	4.0	1	4.0
Perceived barrier								
It is difficult to find time to plan healthy meals because of school commitments	13	52.0	10	40.0	14	56.0	11	44.0
Strongly Agree	5	20.0	9	36.0	8	32.0	10	40.0
Agree	6	24.0	4	16.0	1	4.0	4	16.0
Disagree	1	4.0	2	8.0	2	8.0	0	0.0
Strongly disagree								

Assessing the respondents' severity/seriousness of the effect of unhealthy eating practices on their health, it was found that while more than half (56%) of the respondents in the NE alone group disagreed that they think there is nothing wrong in eating lots of salt and sugar, fewer respondents disagreed in the NE&MTM and MTM alone group at 32% and 28% respectively. Furthermore, there were 3%, 36%, 32% and 36% of the respondents in the NE&MTM group, NE alone group, MTM alone group and control group respectively who disagreed that taking soft drink as often as possible will not result into health consequences now or later in life.

Assessing the respondents' benefit of eating healthy on health, it was found that more than half of the respondents in the NE alone and MTM alone groups at 52% and 56% respectively disagreed that they do not think that healthy food can prevent diseases. Also, fewer respondents strongly agreed that consuming a healthy diet will help in lowering their cholesterol level in the NE&MTM group (12%), NE alone group (8%) and control group (16%). Furthermore, more than half of respondents in the control group (56%), MTM alone group (56%) and NE&MTM group (56%) agreed that a healthy diet reduced their risk of developing cardiovascular diseases.

Assessing the respondents' barrier towards healthy eating, it was found that a larger proportion of respondents in across all four groups (NE&MTM-52%; NE alone-40%; MTM alone-56% and Control-44%) strongly agreed that it is difficult to find time to plan healthy meals because of school commitments.

Effect of nutrition education and mobile text messages on respondents' perceived susceptibility, severity and benefit

The change in the level of perceived susceptibility of the effect of unhealthy eating practices on health between baseline and the 8-weeks follow up indicated a mean differences of 2.696, 3.458, 1.000 and 0.739 for the nutrition education and mobile text messages group, nutrition education alone, mobile text messages alone and control group respectively (see Table 3). The observed difference in means of nutrition education and mobile text messages group and nutrition education alone was statistically significant ($p < 0.05$). However, the observed difference in means of mobile text messages group and control group was not statistically significant ($p > 0.05$) (see Table 3). The result indicated that the nutrition education alone group had a greater change in respondent level of perceived susceptibility of the effect of unhealthy eating practices on health between baseline and the 8-weeks follow up (see Table 3).

The change in the level of perceived severity/seriousness of the effect of unhealthy eating practices on health between baseline and the 8-weeks follow up indicated a mean differences of 2.652, 2.792, 3.167 and 0.217 for the nutrition education and mobile text messages group, nutrition education alone, mobile text messages alone and control group respectively (see Table 3). The observed difference in means in all the experimental groups across these periods were statistically significant ($p < 0.05$) (See Table 3). However, the variation observed in the control group was not statistically significant ($p > 0.05$). The result further indicated that the mobile text messages group alone had a greater change in respondent level of perceived severity/seriousness of the effect of unhealthy eating practices on health between baseline and the 8-weeks follow up (see Table 3).

The change in the level of perceived benefits of eating healthy on health between baseline and the 8-weeks follow up indicated a mean differences of 2.304, 2.292, 0.958 and 0.261 for the nutrition education and mobile text messages group, nutrition education alone, mobile text messages alone and control group respectively (see Table 3). The observed difference in means of nutrition education and mobile text messages group and nutrition education alone was statistically significant ($p < 0.05$). However, the observed difference in means of mobile text messages group and control group was not statistically significant ($p > 0.05$) (see Table 3). The result indicated that the nutrition education alone group had a greater change in respondent level of perceived benefits of eating healthy on health between baseline and the 8-weeks follow up (see Table 3).

Table 3. Paired Sample T-test showing the paired differences between the respondents' perception at baseline and 8-weeks follow-up

Variables: Perceived Susceptibility	N	Maximum points on scale of measure	Baseline		8 weeks' follow-up		Mean difference	df	t	P-value
			x̄(SE)	±SD	x̄(SE)	±SD				
Nutrition education and Mobile text messages	23									
Baseline vs 8-weeks follow up		18	10.43(0.94)	4.53	13.13(0.57)	2.73	2.696	22	2.362	0.027
Nutrition education alone	24									
Baseline vs 8-weeks follow up		18	8.79(0.68)	3.37	12.25(0.72)	3.52	3.458	23	3.830	0.001
Mobile text messages alone	24									
Baseline vs 8-weeks follow up		18	9.75(0.77)	3.79	10.75(0.68)	3.36	1.000	23	1.004	0.326
Control	23									
Baseline vs 8-weeks follow up		18	8.30(0.70)	3.36	9.04(0.68)	3.26	0.739	22	0.690	0.497
Variable: Perceived Severity/Seriousness		**Maximum points on scale of measure**	**Baseline**		**8weeks' follow-up**		**Mean difference**	**df**	**t**	**P-value**
			x̄(SE)	±SD	x̄(SE)	±SD				
Nutrition education and Mobile text messages	23									
Baseline vs 8-weeks follow up		18	11.08(0.86)	4.14	13.73(0.52)	2.50	2.652	22	2.352	0.028
Nutrition education alone	24									
Baseline vs 8-weeks follow up		18	9.08(0.811)	3.97	11.87(0.66)	3.26	2.792	23	2.762	0.011
Mobile text messages alone	24									
Baseline vs 8-weeks follow up		18	7.95(0.74)	3.65	11.12(0.68)	3.37	3.167	23	3.771	0.001

Table 3. (Continued)

Variables: Perceived Susceptibility	N	Maximum points on scale of measure	Baseline		8 weeks' follow-up		Mean difference	df	t	P-value
Control	23									
Baseline vs 8-weeks follow up		18	7.65(0.75)	3.61	7.86(0.73)	3.54	0.217	22	0.273	0.778
Variable: Perceived Benefit		**Maximum points on scale of measure**	**Baseline**		**8weeks' follow-up**		**Mean difference**	**df**	**t**	**P-value**
			x̄(SE)	±SD	x̄(SE)	±SD				
Nutrition education and Mobile text messages	23									
Baseline vs 8-weeks follow up		18	9.04(0.62)	3.00	11.34(0.59)	2.85	2.304	22	2.635	0.015
Nutrition education alone	24									
Baseline vs 8-weeks follow up		18	11.25(0.55)	2.73	13.54(0.53)	2.63	2.292	23	2.803	0.010
Mobile text messages alone	24									
Baseline vs 8-weeks follow up		18	10.12(0.49)	2.40	11.08(0.54)	2.66	0.958	23	1.166	0.256
Control	23									
Baseline vs 8-weeks follow up		18	9.69(0.58)	2.80	9.95(0.54)	2.61	0.261	22	0.350	0.729

p-value obtained by t-test.
significant at $p<0.05$.

Effect of nutrition education and mobile text messages on respondents' eating practice

At baseline, the practice of healthy eating was measured on a 54-point rating scale. At baseline, the mean score for control group was 23.21 ± 3.02, the NE&MTM group was 23.34 ± 3.22, the NE alone group was 22.91 ± 4.50 and the MTM alone group was 20.75 ± 4.92. At endline, level of practice of good dietary pattern were also measured on a 54-point rating scale. At endline, results showed that there was a significant increase in the eating practices of participants in the experimental groups between baseline and 8-weeks follow-up (NE and MTM $\bar{x}$=31.26±6.74, mean diff.=7.913, t_{22}=4.778, p=0.000; NE $\bar{x}$=28.04±5.42, mean diff.=5.12, t_{23}=3.360, p=0.003; MPC $\bar{x}$=25.12±5.17, mean diff.=4.375, t_{23}=3.498, p=0.002). For control group there was no significant difference in respondents eating practices between baseline and 8-weeks follow-up ($\bar{x}$=23.21±3.02, $\bar{x}$=23.34±2.93, mean diff.=0.13, t_{22}=0.175, p=0.863) (see Table 4).

Table 4. Impact evaluation of intervention on eating practice between baseline and 8 weeks' follow-up

Group		**Baseline**		**8 weeks Post-intervention**		**Mean difference**	**df**	**t**	**P-value**
		x̄ (SE)	±SD	x̄ (SE)	±SD				
Control	23	23.21(0.63)	3.02	23.34(0.61)	2.93	0.130	22	0.175	0.863
NE&MTM	23	23.34(0.67)	3.22	31.26(1.40)	6.74	7.913	23	4.778	0.000
NE alone	24	22.91(0.91)	4.50	28.04(1.10)	5.42	5.125	23	3.360	0.003
MTM alone	24	20.75(0.98)	4.92	25.12(1.05)	5.17	4.375	22	3.498	0.002

p-value obtained by t-test.
significant at p<0.05.

Conclusion

Findings from studies conducted among undergraduate students in different Nigerian states lend credence to the growing epidemic; the reported prevalence of overweight and obesity among undergraduate in Abia state was 19.5% and 8.9%(7); 32.8% and 6.3% in Lagos state (8); 15.1% and 3.5% in Ogun state (9); 8.82% and 17.45% in Oyo state respectively (10). Compared to other developed regions of the world, the reported prevalence of obesity among young adult in Nigeria is low however; this is rapidly increasing due to the corresponding rise in the behavioural antecedent risk factors specifically unhealthy diets (11).

Poor dietary practices such as unhealthy dieting, meal skipping, fast food consumption, poor food choices, unhealthy snaking and consumption of sugary drinks have been observed among respondents in this study. As university students develop autonomy in their food choices, many struggle with eating a healthful diet in school (12). For many Nigerian students the day is not complete without observing the "daily ritual" of visiting a fast food joint and most of the fast food restaurants in the cities have begun to open centres within and very close to schools especially university campuses.

Respondents practices poor eating habit, propounded by the high intake of carbonated drinks, fast food and low intake of fruits and vegetables; Availability and accessibility to healthy food choices was a major barrier against adoption of healthy eating habit among respondents. Many factors have been reported to influence the unhealthy eating practices of young adults, which include individual and environmental factors (13). Another study (14) also found out that the personal factors are hectic lifestyles (leaving little time for shopping and cooking), taste preferences, negative attitudes and perceived norms regarding healthy eating, and lack of knowledge, skills, self-efficacy and social support. Studies has also shown that one major reinforcing factors contributing to unhealthy dietary practice of young adults is peer influence.

The combination of both nutrition education and mobile text messages however improved respondents' healthy eating practice, this more significantly than isolation of nutrition education and mobile text messages interventions separately. Availability and accessibility to healthy food choices is beyond an individual's control, putting the charge on the institution bodies. Stakeholders within the institutions have key roles to play in enhancing positive healthy eating habit in controlling the food chain structure within its confinement. Regulation of food items sold within the campus will play a huge role in reduction in the barriers of accessing these healthy food items, more so at a more reduced cost.

ACKNOWLEDGMENTS

To my supervisor, professor Ademola Amosu, thank you for your time and guidance during the course of this research. I also wish to express my sincere thanks to the Babcock University for accepting me into the graduate program and for creating the platform for academic excellence. I am grateful to all the schools involved in this study for their maximum cooperation and support given to me along the way. A very special gratitude goes out to my parents for helping and providing the funding for the work. Lastly, special thanks to Almighty God for seeing me through the course of this project. This study was self-sponsored. The authors declare that they have no conflict of interest. Informed consent was obtained from each individual participant involved in this study. This study was conducted in accordance with the 1964 Declaration of Helsinki and its subsequent amendments. No animal was involved in this study.

REFERENCES

[1] Fabian C, Pagan I, Rios JL, Betancourt J, Cruz SY, González AM, et al. Dietary patterns and their association with sociodemographic characteristics and perceived

academic stress of college students in Puerto Rico. P R Health Sci J 2013;32(1):36-43.

[2] Freedman MR. Development, evaluation, and validation of environmental assessment tools to evaluate the college nutrition environment. J Am Coll Health 2010;58(6):565-68.

[3] Russell-Mayhew S, McVey G, Bardick A, Ireland A. Mental health, wellness, and childhood overweight/obesity. J Obes 2012;11:281-87.

[4] Ezezika O, Oh J, Edeagu N, Boyo W. Gamification of nutrition: a preliminary study on the impact of gamification on nutrition knowledge, attitude, and behaviour of adolescents in Nigeria. Nutr Health 2018;24(3):137-44.

[5] Otuneye AT, Ahmed PA, Abdulkarim AA, Aluko OO, Shatima DR. Relationship between dietary habits and nutritional status among adolescents in Abuja municipal area council of Nigeria. Niger J Paediatr 2017;44(3):128-35.

[6] Curbing N. Noncommunicable diseases in africa: youth are key to curbing the epidemic and achieving sustainable development. Washington, DC: Population Reference Bureau, 2015.

[7] Ejike CE, Ijeh II. Obesity in young-adult Nigerians: variations in prevalence determined by anthropometry and bioelectrical impedance analysis, and the development of % body fat prediction equations. Int Arch Med 2012;5(1):22.

[8] Olatona FA, Onabanjo OO, Ugbaja RN, Nnoaham KE, Adelekan DA. Dietary habits and metabolic risk factors for non-communicable diseases in a university undergraduate population. J Health Popul Nutr 2018;37(1):21.

[9] Oladoyinbo C, Fadipe Y, Sobo A. Dietary habits and portion sizes associated with overweight and obesity among undergraduate students in Ogun state, Nigeria (P04-184-19). Curr Dev Nutr 2019;3:51-4.

[10] Olatunbosun ST, Kaufman JS, Bella AF. Prevalence of obesity and overweight in urban adult Nigerians. Obes Rev 2011;12(4):233-41.

[11] Oluwasanu MM, Oladepo O. Effects of a multi-level intervention on the pattern of physical activity among in-school adolescents in Oyo state Nigeria: a cluster randomised trial. BMC Public Health 2017;17(1):833.

[12] Cluskey M, Grobe D. College weight gain and behavior transitions: male and female differences. J Am Nutr Diet 2009;109(2):325-9.

[13] Eleojo AA, Charles UC, Anyebe JM. Physical Activity Level and Dietary Pattern of Undergraduate Students of Kogi state University, Anyigba Kogi state. ACRI 2019;21:1-8.

[14] Schätzer M, Rust P, Elmadfa I. Fruit and vegetable intake in Austrian adults: intake frequency, serving sizes, reasons for and barriers to consumption, and potential for increasing consumption. Public Health Nutr 2010;13(4):480-7.

In: Pediatrics and Adolescent Health ISBN: 978-1-68507-490-6
Editors: J. Merrick and M. Morad

Chapter 16

THE CONSUMPTION OF MILK, VEGETABLES AND FRUITS, FISH, WHOLEMEAL BREAD AND FAST FOOD MEALS AMONG 15-YEAR-OLD TEENAGERS DEPENDING ON THE BMI VALUE

Wioletta Waksmańska**, PhD, Rafał Bobiński, PhD, Renata Łukasik, PhD and Anna Pielesz, PhD

Faculty of Health Sciences and Faculty of Materials,
Civil and Environmental Engineering,
University of Bielsko-Biala,
Bielsko-Biala, Poland

* Corresponding Author's E-mail: wwaksmanska@ath.bielsko.pl.

ABSTRACT

The objective of this chapter was to evaluate the relationship between eating habits and BMI values in 15-year-old teenagers. The studies covered pupils of third grades of the middle school. Energetic and nutrient requirements were determined for each child individually. The number of daily calorie intake was determined with the use of the DIETA FAO. The obtained average consumption values were compared with nutrition norms of US Department of Agriculture. Obesity was noted in the group of girls, in the group of boys there were instances only of overweight. All children consumed at least three meals a day. No more than 50% of the respondents consumed an afternoon snack. Milk was drunk every day by 50% of boys with excessive body weight, while 75% of them ate vegetables and fruit only once a week. Fish usually appeared in the menu once or two-three times a week. Fast food products were consumed by all respondents. The analysis demonstrated that the amount of time spent in front of the computer had a statistically significant impact on body weight in the case of boys. In the group of girls the time a second breakfast was consumed was statistically significant. Eating habits of middle-school students are not in line with nutrition principles - intake of milk, fish, vegetables and fruit is insufficient. It is necessary to take educational action addressed at youth and their caregivers.

INTRODUCTION

The occurrence of improper body weight values, particularly overweight and obesity, has psychological and social implications. It is also a serious public health problem. Excessive body weight is very often caused by contemporary lifestyle (1, 2). The main role in the pathogenesis of abnormal body weight values is played by genetic and environmental factors, and by behavior (3). Health behavior is one of the most important factors determining health - it starts to develop in early childhood and is transferred into adult life (4). An important element of the health behavior are food preferences, out of which the most important are daily consumption of sweetened beverages, consumption of food containing high amounts of fats, excessive consumption of energy, and low intake of fruit and vegetables. Food preferences constitute an important factor influencing the occurrence of excessive body weight which poses the risk of developing arterial hypertension, type 2 diabetes or dyslipidemia in young school-aged people. Excessive body weight occurring throughout school is maintained until adulthood (2, 5-6). Food preferences, leading to improper balancing of diet, despite appropriate energy value of consumed meals, may lead to nutritional deficiencies (e.g., lack of vitamins). Consuming cakes, donuts and crisps as well as drinking sweetened beverages exposes youth to the risk of malnutrition (7). At the same time, nutritional disorders may result from the aspiration to have a "perfect body" (5). Teenagers of middle school age go through the period of emotional development in which personal identity is formed and, simultaneously, in which activities that are risky for health are undertaken. Therefore, school becomes an important place for educational activities aimed at creating pupils' personal values (2, 8-9).

Per study

The objective of the study was to evaluate the frequency of occurrence of abnormal BMI values and the influence of eating habits on BMI values in 15-year-old teenagers.

GATHERING AND ASSESSMENT OF ANTHROPOMETRIC DATA

The study was conducted in one of common middle schools in southern Poland in February 2017. The studies covered all pupils of third grades of the middle school. Participation in the study was voluntary. Consent to conduct the study has been obtained from the children and their caregivers. The study covered the total of 133 15-year-old pupils (57 girls and 76 boys). All children were subject to the measurements of body weight, body height and BMI. The BMI value was classified according to the WHO and the US Department of Health and Human Services and US Department of Agriculture recommendations: BMI below 5th percentile - underweight, BMI between 5th and 85th percentile - normal body weight, BMI between 85th - 95th percentile - overweight and BMI above 95th percentile – obesity (10, 11). While determining physical activity the following activities were included: physical education classes (compulsory) and extracurricular physical activities such as team sports (football, volleyball, etc.), dance classes (contemporary dance), swimming.

Gathering and assessment of food intake data

The questionnaire concerning daily food consumption for the period of seven years was filled in with assistance of the person conducting the survey. In order to determine the number of calories consumed, the size of the portion was verified with the use of "The album of photographs of food products and dishes" (12). The number of daily calorie intake was determined with the use of the DIETA FAO program containing data about 1,067 typical food products. A detailed description of the study was included in an earlier publication (13). Energetic and nutrient requirements were determined for each child individually. The obtained average consumption values were compared with nutrition norms of United States Department of Agriculture for people who are moderately physically active with *nutrition norms for Polish population* (11, 14). Energy requirements for the analyzed population was determined according to the following norm: 2,600-2,700 kcal/24 hours for boys and 2,100-2,200 kcal/24 hours for girls with low or moderate physical activity.

Statistical analysis

Analyses were performed in the programs PQStat 1.6.4; PSPP 0.10.4; MS Office 2013 (RS for Excel), "R." Analyzed variables were measured on both nominal and quantitative scales. In all analyses the level of significance was set at < 0.05. Normal distribution of continuous variables was verified using the Shapiro-Wilk's W test. In the case the nature of variables differed from a normal one, a non-parametric Kruskal–Wallis test was used. In the case of qualitative variables an $\chi 2$ test was applied, and if it failed to meet the test objectives – a precise Fisher's test.

Bioethics committee permission

The study was approved by the Bioethics Review Board of Bielsko-Biala (No: 2017/06/1/4) which is in accordance with the Declaration of Helsinki. All participants gave their informed consent for taking part in the research, the participation in this study was voluntary and the anonymity of participants was preserved.

FINDINGS

The conducted analysis demonstrated the occurrence of low body weight in 20.3% of the respondents who most frequently were girls. Obesity was noted in the group of girls, in the group of boys there were no instances of obesity, only of overweight. Altogether, overweight occurred in 12.8% of all respondents. All children consumed at least three meals a day. A second breakfast was a common meal. 61% of girls and 67% of boys ate a second breakfast. No more than 50% of the respondents consumed an afternoon snack. The statistically significant impact on the BMI value had the frequency of eating breakfast - in the group of girls it was the second breakfast, while in the boys group it was the first breakfast (see Table 1).

The time of eating meals varied greatly. Breakfast was eaten at 6 a.m. at the earliest. Boys with normal and excessive body weight and girls with normal body weight ate supper very late, at 10 p.m. (see Table 2).

In the tested group the largest amount of time in front of the computer was spent by girls with excessive body weight (195 minutes/day) and boys with underweight (255 minutes/day). All pupils participated in physical education classes at school for 135 minutes/week. The rest of the time devoted to physical activity was in the form of organized classes (dance, football, volleyball classes). The most active were boys with normal body weight who spent an average of 445 minutes per week on physical activities. A similar amount of physical activity (440 minutes/week) was observed in the case of girls with normal body weight. In the group of girls the time devoted to physical activity had a statistically significant and positive impact on the BMI value – the longer the time, the lower the body weight. In the group of boys the same impact had the time spent in front of the computer – the shorter the time, the lower BMI value (see Table 3).

While analyzing the frequency of milk, vegetables and fruit consumption, it was observed that a large group of pupils, both boys and girls, consumed these products 2-3 times per week. Milk was drunk every day by 50% of boys with excessive body weight, while 75% of them ate vegetables and fruit only once a week. The frequency of fruit and vegetable intake had a statistically significant and positive impact on the BMI value (see Table 4).

Table 1. Frequency of meals in the analyzed group considering body mass and sex

Sex	Frequency of consuming meals	Underweight		Normal body weight		Overweight		Total		Test statistic
		n	%	n	%	n	%	n	%	Pearson chi-square
Girls	I breakfast	13	100%	36	100%	8	100%	57	100%	$\chi 2$ (df=2) – 5.2
	II breakfast	7	54%	23	64%	5	63%	35	61%	$\chi 2$ (df=2) – 11.4*
	Dinner	13	100%	36	100%	8	100%	57	100%	$\chi 2$ (df=2) – 5.5
	Afternoon snack	5	38%	18	50%	4	50%	27	47%	$\chi 2$ (df=2) – 0.26
	Supper	13	100%	36	100%	8	100%	57	100%	$\chi 2$ (df=2) – 6.15
Boys	I breakfast	14	100%	50	100%	12	100%	76	100%	$\chi 2$ (df=2) – 10.82*
	II breakfast	8	57%	38	76%	5	42%	51	67%	$\chi 2$ (df=2) – 1.25
	Dinner	14	100%	50	100%	12	100%	76	100%	$\chi 2$ (df=2) – 3.42
	Afternoon snack	6	43%	22	44%	3	25%	31	41%	$\chi 2$ (df=2) – 1.21
	Supper	14	100%	50	100%	12	100%	76	100%	$\chi 2$ (df=2) – 3.43

*$p < 0.05$.

Table 2. Presentation of eating hours in the analyzed group, taking into account body weight and sex

Meal time		Underweight			Normal body weight			Overweight		
		Earliest	Latest	Median	Earliest	Latest	Median	Earliest	Latest	Median
Girls	I breakfast	6:00	10:00	7:00	6:00	10:00	7:00	6:00	9:00	7:00
	II breakfast	10:00	12:00	11:00	10:00	12:00	10:00	11:00	12:00	11:00
	Dinner	14:00	16:00	14:00	12:00	17:00	15:00	14:00	16:00	15:00
	Afternoon snack	15:00	19:00	17:00	15:00	19:00	17:00	16:00	18:00	17:00
	Supper	19:00	21:00	20:00	17:00	22:00	19:00	18:00	20:00	19:00
Boys	I breakfast	6:00	9:00	7:00	6:00	10:00	7:00	6:00	10:00	7:00
	II breakfast	10:00	12:00	10:00	8:00	12:00	10:00	9:00	12:00	11:00
	Dinner	13:00	17:00	14:00	12:00	17:00	15:00	12:00	17:00	15:00
	Afternoon snack	16:00	19:00	17:00	16:00	19:00	17:00	15:00	19:00	17:00
	Supper	18:00	21:00	20:00	18:00	22:00	20:00	17:00	22:00	19:00

Table 3. Time spent in front of the computer and on physical activities in the analyzed group, considering body mass and sex

The number of minutes spent in front of the computer and devoted to physical activity		Underweight			Normal body weight			Overweight			Test statistic
		Min	Max	Average	Min	Max	Average	Min	Max	Average	Pearson chi-square
Girls	Time spent in front of the computer/day	30	600	170	60	600	175	60	300	195	χ2 (df=2) – 5.93
	Physical activity/week	135	480	340	135	960	440	135	360	285	χ2 (df=2) – 13.21*
Boys	Time spent in front of the computer/day	120	480	255	60	600	205	60	360	205	χ2 (df=2) – 9.29*
	Physical activity/week	135	600	395	135	1080	445	135	480	375	χ2 (df=2) – 3.3

*$p < 0.05$.

Table 4. Frequency of milk, vegetables and fruit intake in the studied group, including body mass and sex

Frequency of intake Body mass/Sex		Every day		2-3 times a week		Once a week		2-3 times a month		Test statistic Pearson chi-square
		n	%	n	%	n	%	n	%	
Milk										
Boys	Underweight	4	28.6%	6	42.8%	-		4	28.6%	χ2 (df=2) – 3.47
	Normal body weight	13	26%	25	50%	12	24%	-		
	Overweight	6	50%	4	33.3%	1	8.4%	1	8.4%	
Girls	Underweight	2	15.4%	7	53.8%	4	30.8%	-		χ2 (df=2) – 2.07
	Normal body weight	14	38.8%	12	33.5%	10	27.7%	-		
	Overweight	3	37.5%	3	37.5%	2	25%	-		

Table 4. (Continued)

Frequency of intake Body mass/Sex		Every day		2-3 times a week		Once a week		2-3 times a month		Test statistic Pearson chi-square
		n	%	n	%	n	%	n	%	
Vegetables and fruit										
Boys	Underweight	5	35.7%	8	57.1%	1	7.2%	-		$\chi 2$ (df=2) =48.15*
	Normal body weight	8	16%	37	74%	5	10%	-		
	Overweight	1	8.4%	2	16.6%	9	75%	-		
Girls	Underweight	1	7.7%	12	92.3%	-		-		$\chi 2$ (df=2) =64.57*
	Normal body weight	8	22.2%	25	69.4%	3	8.4%	-		
	Overweight	1	12.5%	6	75%	1	12.5%	-		

*$p < 0.05$.

Table 5. Frequency of fish, wholemeal bread and fast food intake in the studied group, including body mass and sex

Frequency of intake Body mass/Sex		Every day		2-3 times a week		Once a week		2-3 times a month		Once a month		Test statistic Pearson chi-square
		n	%	n	%	n	%	n	%	n	%	
Fish												
Boys	Underweight	-		4	28.6%	2	14.3%	8	57.1%	-		$\chi 2$ (df=2) =19.55*
	Normal body weight	-		8	16%	33	66%	4	8%	5	10%	
	Overweight	-		4	33.3%	2	16.7%	2	16.7%	4	33.3%	

Frequency of intake Body mass/Sex		Every day		2-3 times a week		Once a week		2-3 times a month		Once a month		Test statistic Pearson chi-square
		n	%	n	%	n	%	n	%	n	%	
Girls	Underweight	-		4	30.8%	5	38.4%	4	30.8%	-		$\chi2$ (df=2) =30.49*
	Normal body weight	-		14	38.8%	10	27.7%	12	33.5%	-		
	Overweight	-		-		3	37.5%	5	62.5%	-		
Wholemeal bread												
Boys	Underweight	2	14.2%	4	28.6%	4	28.6%	4	28.6%	-		$\chi2$ (df=2) =5.09
	Normal body weight	15	30%	9	18%	12	24%	14	28%	-		
	Overweight	3	25%	4	33.3%	4	33.3%	1	8.4%	-		
Girls	Underweight	2	15.4%	2	15.4%	1	7.7%	7	53.8%	1	7.7%	$\chi2$ (df=2) =5.44
	Normal body weight	11	30.5%	9	25%	6	16.7%	7	19.4%	3	8.4%	
	Overweight	2	25%	1	12.5%	2	25%	2	25%	1	12.5%	
Fast food meals												
Boys	Underweight	-		-		4	28.6%	1	7.1%	9	64.3%	$\chi2$ (df=2) – 29.02*
	Normal body weight	-		2	4%	12	24%	7	14%	29	58%	
	Overweight	2	16.8%	3	25.2%	5	41.2%	2	16.8%	-		
Girls	Underweight	-		-		1	7.7%	3	23.1%	9	69.2%	$\chi2$ (df=2) =44.07*
	Normal body weight	-		1	2.8%	7	19.4%	8	22.2%	20	55.6%	
	Overweight	-		3	37.5%	3	37.5%	2	25%	-		

*$p < 0.05$.

Table 6. Median of calories intake per day and percentage of norm coverage

Sex	Underweight		Normal body weight		Overweight		Test statistic
	Energy kcal	% norm	Energy kcal	% norm	Energy kcal	% norm	Pearson chi-square
Boys	2 671.9	100%	2 572.8	97%	3 385.2	128%	$\chi2$ (df=2) = 60.29*
Girls	1 659.6	77%	2 143.2	100%	3 075.7	143%	$\chi2$ (df=2) = 89.99*

*p < 0.05.

Table 7. Relation between body mass and selected eating habits in the analyzed group broken down according to sex

Analyzed variable	Test result					
	Underweight		Normal body weight		Overweight	
	Normal body weight	Overweight	Underweight	Overweight	Underweight	Normal body weight
Boys						
Time spent in front of the computer/day	5.993*	9.825*	5.993*	3.425	9.825*	3.425
Energy	1.251	22.522*	1.251	29.022*	22.522*	29.022*
Fast food meals	3.476	9.775*	3.476	9.875*	9.775*	9.875*
Girls						
II breakfast time	0.211	1.649	0.211	11.400*	1.649	11.400*
Physical activity/week	13.219*	4.605	13.219*	18.47 *	4.605	18.47 *
Energy	79.997*	86.997*	79.997*	96.997*	86.997*	96.997*
Fast food meals	9.775*	13.825*	9.775*	11.800*	13.825*	11.800*

*p < 0.05.

Fish usually appeared in the menu once or two-three times a week. A large group of boys with excessive body weight (33.3%) ate fish occasionally once a month. The statistically significant relationship was demonstrated between the frequency of the consumption of fish and the BMI value. Circa 30% of the teenagers with normal body weight stated that wholemeal bread was included in their daily diet, and in the case of more than 50% of girls with underweight wholemeal bread was eaten only 2-3 times a month. Fast food products (pizza, hamburgers, chips) were consumed by all respondents. They were eaten every day by two boys with excessive body weight, while they were eaten more rarely (once a month) by the teenagers with underweight. There is also a small group of respondents with normal body weight (2.8 - 4%) that consumed fast food products 2-3 times a week. The frequent consumption of fast food meals had a negative impact on the BMI value (see Table 5). Daily caloric value of consumed food was within the normal range in a group of girls and boys with normal body weight and in the group of boys with underweight. The differences in calorie intake in both boys and girls were statistically significant (see Table 6). The analysis demonstrated that the amount of time spent in front of the computer had a statistically significant impact on body weight in the case of boys. In the group of girls the time a second breakfast was consumed and the amount of time devoted to physical activity was statistically significant. A statistically significant correlation between body weight, the amount of daily calorie intake and fast food product consumption was observed in the group of both boys and girls (see Table 7).

DISCUSSION

Improper body weight values are caused by the lack of balance between calorie consumption and energy expenditure. Studies have shown that the occurrence of overweight and obesity constantly increases (1). While studying a group of Polish 13-16-year-old teenagers Czajka and co-authors (15) demonstrated the occurrence of excessive body weight in 21% of girls and 25.6% of boys. Results of the studies (NHANES) conducted in the years 2013-2014 showed that circa 16.2% of children and adolescents in the United States are overweight and another 17.2% are obese (16). The WHO studies conducted in the years 2009-2010 proved that overweight and obesity concern 10-23% of 15-year-old people (17). The percentage of youth with overweight and obesity is much higher in Saudi Arabia. In the group of 14-16-year-old teenagers 31.5% are overweight and 45% are obese (6).

In the authors' own research such frequent occurrence of excessive body weight was not observed. However, there were more frequent instances of body mass insufficiency which concerned 20.3% of the tested group. In 2007 the occurrence of the BMI value below 5th percentile concerned 16% of teenagers in Saudi Arabia (6). The study conducted by Czajka and co-authors demonstrated more frequent occurrence of body-weight deficiency in girls than in boys (15). The reason of body-weight deficiency is consuming too low-calorie meals (18). The analysis of the authors' own materials confirmed this correlation with reference to girls with underweight whose meals included 1660 kilo-calories per day. Body weight disorders result, inter alia, from the lack of a healthy lifestyle, of which time devoted to physical activity is an important element. According to guidelines released by the US Department of Health and Human Services the activity should amount to 60 minutes per day, i.e., 420 minutes per week (11). Asked about physical activities, teenagers most frequently listed participating in physical education classes at school. According to Starczewska (5) the situation concerns more than 80% of teenagers. In the authors' own research it was observed that all of the middle school pupils participated in physical education classes which amounted to 135 minutes per week. It was also noted that the group of teenagers with normal body weight was the most active. The least active were pupils with excessive body weight who, at the same time, spent the largest amount of time in front of the computer. In the group of boys the time spent in front of the computer had a statistically significant effect on body weight. It confirms the fact that overweight and obesity more often refer to people with a sedentary lifestyle and who spend a lot of time in front of the TV. At the same time, watching TV fosters sneaking high-calorie products (crisps, sweetened drinks) and causes further gain of body weight (19).

Dietary recommendations indicate the necessity to consume four to five meals per day (11, 14, 17, 20). The analysis of the authors' own material demonstrated that in the groups of both girls and boys at least three meals per day were consumed. In both tested groups five meals per day were consumed with the same frequency (81.6%). According to Szczepańska's study conducted on a group of Polish and Czech middle school youth 4-5 meals per day are present in the diet of 45.5% of the Polish teenagers and 48.5% of the Czech teenagers (21). A first breakfast is an important component of the diet. The lack of a first breakfast may lead to increased risk of obesity and decline in psycho-physical activity of a child (14, 19). In the group of Czech middle school teenagers breakfast was part of daily diet in 42.6% of case (21). The authors' own research did not confirm this result because all of the tested pupils declared they ate a first breakfast every day. However, it was observed that the time of a second breakfast consumption had a statistically significant effect on BMI of girls with excessive body weight.

According to recommendations of the US Department of Health and Human Services and US Department of Agriculture the time of meals is important as well as consuming several portions of vegetables and fruit, and 3-4 glasses of milk per day. A first breakfast should be eaten before leaving home, whereas supper 2-3 hours before bedtime (11). According to the authors' own research the time of meals varied, however, a first breakfast was most often consumed at 7 a.m., that is before leaving home for school. In the case of supper teenagers sometimes consumed a meal at 10 p.m., which is definitely too late. Szczepanska and co-authors (21) demonstrated that breakfast before leaving home was eaten by 57.4% of the pupils and only 44.4% of them had supper 2-3 hours before bedtime.

Daily consumption of milk is not a dietary preference typical of middle school teenagers. Middle school pupils from Lublin stated that milk and its products were included in a diet in 37.3% of cases, yet in more than 29% of cases milk was only an addition to other breakfast products (22). In the authors' own research it was observed that milk was drunk every day by boys with excessive body weight and girls with normal body weight, almost one-third of boys with underweight drank milk only 2-3 times a month. While conducting an analysis of eating habits Szczepańska and co-authors divided the tested group according to body weight (underweight, norm, overweight and obesity) and showed that milk and milk drinks were consumed at least once a day by 58.3% of the tested people with underweight and by 51.7% of the ones with overweight and obesity. However, the tested group was comprised of the youth from all middle school and high school levels, no distinction was made with regard to the sex of the tested pupils (23). This could have significantly affected the study results as eating habits of pupils from the first level of middle school may be totally different than the ones of pupils from the third level of high school. In order to eliminate such errors the authors' own research focused on a group of students of the same age.

According to US Department of Health and Human Services and US Department of Agriculture, consumption of dairy products, vegetables and fruit among American teenagers is insufficient (11). According to Polish studies, vegetables were included in the daily diet of only 13.6% of middle school pupils (22). The middle school pupils' diet included more fruit, consuming it several times a day or every day, depending on the region covered by the research (4-6, 20-21). The analysis of the authors' own material demonstrated that in most cases teenagers consumed vegetables and fruit several times a week. Boys with excessive body weight ate vegetables and fruit the most rarely.

Worse results were obtained after the analysis of the frequency of consuming fish. In most cases fish was consumed 1-2 times a week. A large group of middle school children ate fish only occasionally, that is once a month. Consumption of wholemeal bread was at the same level, it appeared in the diet up to four times a week (20-21). The authors' own research confirmed insufficient consumption of fish. In the case of wholemeal bread - it was eaten by 25% of the teenagers with excessive body weight and by 30% of the ones with normal body weight. According to the study conducted by Stankiewicz and co-authors, girls are more likely to eat wholemeal bread than boys (24). Both wholemeal bread and fish constitute an important part of diet owing to their nutritional values.

Fast food appears in the diet more often than fish and wholemeal bread. Each middle school student eats pizza, chips or hamburgers. The authors' own research demonstrated that fast food products affected the tested pupils' body weight. 4% of Polish middle school students ate this type of products a few times a day and 3.6% of the students consumed them every day (21-22). In the city of Rijad students ate fast food an average of 4.5 times per week (6) Fast food products, like highly processed food, are characterized by low price, attractive packaging and taste, and - at the same time - big portions. In addition, a number of advertisements suggesting high content of nutrients may make buying this type of food more frequent (19).

Abnormal eating habits acquired during the juvenile period solidify and continue during adult life increasing the risk of metabolic syndrome, arterial hypertension, diabetes, asthma, arthritis or kidney diseases (8, 25). Schools are priority institutions for promoting pro-health activities through education aiming at raising awareness, critical assessment of one's own diet or physical activity and monitoring nutritional status during puberty. Teachers at school do not always possess the necessary knowledge to undertake this type of activities. Therefore, it is crucial to involve health professionals with specialized knowledge in a given discipline to conduct educational activities (2, 24).

CONCLUSION

1. In the analyzed group of youth overweight and obesity were less common than underweight.
2. Eating habits of middle-school students are not in line with nutrition principles - intake of milk, fish, vegetables and fruit is insufficient.

3. Fast food meals, too much time spent in front of the computer and, at the same time, too little time spent on physical activities have a negative influence on body mass.
4. It is necessary to take educational action addressed at youth and their caregivers.

REFERENCES

[1] Gil JM, Takourabt S. Socio-economics, food habits and the prevalence of childhood obesity in Spain. Child Care Health Dev 2016;43(2):250–8.

[2] Schuh DS, Goulart MR, Barbiero SM, Sica CD, Borges R, Moraes DW, Pellanda LC. Healthy school, happy school: Design and protocol for a randomized clinical trial designed to prevent weight gain in children. Arq Bras Cardiol 2017;108(6):501–7.

[3] Wąsowski M, Walicka M, Marcinowska-Suchowierska E. Obesity – definition, epidemiology, pathogenesis. Post Nauk Med 2013;4:301-6.

[4] Ortiz-Hernández L, Gómez-Tello BL. Food consumption in mexican adolescents. Rev Panam Salud Publica 2008;24(2):127-35.

[5] Starczewska M, Tamulewicz A, Stanisławska M, Szkup M, Grochans E, Karakiewicz B. The analysis of selected factors contributing to the health behaviors of teenagers. Fam Med Primary Care Rev 2015;17(1):39–42.

[6] Collison KS, Zaidi MZ, Subhani SN, Al.-Rubeaan K, Shoukri M, Al.-Mohanna FA. Sugar-sweetened carbonated beverage consumption correlates with BMI, waist circumference, and poor dietary choices in school children. BMC Public Health 2010;9(10):234-46.

[7] Steyn N, Eksteen G, Senekal M. Assessment of the dietary intake of schoolchildren in South Africa: 15 Years after the first national study. Nutrients 2016;19(8):1-14.

[8] Decyk-Chęcel A. Children's and adolescents' eating habits. Probl Hig Epidemiol 2017;98(2):103-09.

[9] Siudem A. Risky behaviours of youth at secondary-school age. Psychol Rozwojowa 2013;18(1):69–85.

[10] World Health Organization. Obesity. URL: www.who.int/topics/obesity/en/.

[11] US Department of Health and Human Services and US Department of Agriculture. 2015–2020 dietary guidelines for Americans, 8th edition. URL: http://health.gov/dietaryguidelines/2015/guidelines.

[12] Szponar L, Wolnicka K, Rychlik E. Album of photographs of food products and dishes. Warsaw: National Food and Nutrition Institute, 2010. [Polish]

[13] Waksmańska W, Bobiński R, Ulman-Włodarz I, Pielesz A, Mikulska M. The dietary composition of women who delivered preterm and full-term infants. Appl Nurs Res 2017;35:13–7.

[14] Jarosz M. The standard of nutrition for the Polish population - amendment. Warsaw: National Food and Nutrition Institute,. 2012. [Polish]

[15] Czajka K, Fiszer K, Kołodziej M. The relation between selected health behaviour and body mass index amongst adolescents living in urban and rural areas in south-western Poland. Rocz Panstw Zakl Hig 2013;64(2):135-41.

[16] Ogden CL, Carroll MD, Lawman HG, Fryar CD, Kruszon-Moran D, Kit BK, Flegal KM. Trends in obesity prevalence among children and adolescents in the United States, 1988–1994 through 2013-2014. JAMA 2016;315(21):2292–9.

[17] European Food and Nutrition Action Plan 2015–2020. Copenhagen: WHO Regional Committee for Europe, 2014 Sept 15–18.

[18] World Health Organization. URL: http://www.euro.who.int/__data/assets/pdf_file/0008/253727/64wd14e_FoodNutAP_140426.pdf.

[19] Sitko D, Wojtaś M, Gronowska-Senger A. Food patterns of youth from gymnasium and liceum. Rocz Panstw Zakl Hig 2012;63(3):319-27.

[20] Jarosz M, Wolnicka K, Kłosowska J. Environmental factors associated with prevalence of overweight and obesity among children and adolescents. Post Nauk Med 2011;9:770-7.

[21] Szczepańska E, Deka M, Calyniuk B. Studies to determine nutrition behaviour amongst middle school pupils living in the border areas of Poland and the Czech Republic. Rocz Panstw Zakl Hig 2013;64(3):191-6.

[22] Szczepańska E, Szeja N, Szymkiewicz A, Kowalska A, Lenard B, Bulwicka A. Eating behaviours of middle- and secondary-school pupils from the upper Silesian region in Poland. Rocz Panstw Zakl Hig 2014;65(4):337-44.

[23] Sawicka K, Wawryniuk A, Łuczyk R, Krzyżanowska E, Szubiela N, Łuczyk M, Daniluk J. Assessment of the state of nutritionality and method of food of children of furnishing to basic and gynal schools. J Educ Health Sport 2017;7(7):510-28.

[24] Szczepańska E, Szeja N, Dudzik I, Kołdon A, Jędzura K, Pochopień E, Oleszko M. Eating behaviours and nutrition knowledge of students from selected schools of the upper Silesian region, depending on the body mass index. Nowa Pediatr 2015;2:68-75.

[25] Stankiewicz M, Pieszko M, Śliwińska A, Małgorzewicz S. Obesity and diet awareness among Polish children and adolescents in small towns and villages. Cent Eur J Public Health 2014;22(1):12-6.

[26] Kovesdy CP, Furth S, Zoccali C. Obesity and kidney disease: hidden consequences of the epidemic. Rev Med Chil 2017;145(3):281-91.

In: Pediatrics and Adolescent Health
Editors: J. Merrick and M. Morad
ISBN: 978-1-68507-490-6

Chapter 17

THE ROLE OF GENERAL PRACTITIONERS IN RE-BUILDING WHOLE PERSON WELLNESS OF UNIVERSITY STUDENTS DURING PROTESTS IN HONG KONG: A CASE STUDY

Sze Mon Lo[1,*], Ho Cheong Wong[1], Mei Ho So[1], Birgit Bunzel Linder[2], PhD, Wai Chi Chu[3], PhD and Daniel TL Shek[3], PhD

[1]University Health Services, The Hong Kong Polytechnic University, Hung Hom, Kowloon, Hong Kong
[2]Department of Translation, Lingnan University, Tuen Mun, Hong Kong
[3]Department of Applied Social Sciences, The Hong Kong Polytechnic University, Hung Hom, Kowloon, Hong Kong, PRChina

[*] Corresponding Author's E-mail: dana.lo@polyu.edu.hk.

Abstract

Until the unexpected and prolonged protests that began in June 2019 arising from the Extradition Bill, Hong Kong was recognized as an international city enjoying prosperity and stability. Since then, various studies have shown that the unrest seriously impaired the physical as well as mental well-being of the general public, and particularly of the younger generation who carried most of the movement. In this paper, we present the case of a patient showing surface physical symptoms to illustrate the need for holistic treatment. With reference to the process of traditional Chinese poetry composition, it is argued that beyond the treatment of each physical or mental health symptom, a holistic intervention approach should be adopted to reconstruct whole person wellness. The paper also calls attention to the important role of general medical practitioners in the context of the recent social unrest especially dealing with the aftermath, and argues that a holistic approach results in longer-lasting results for patients with complex issues.

Introduction

In the global context, social unrest occurs in many places including large and affluent cities (such as London and Paris), which creates mental health problems of the general public at large (1). The ongoing "social incident" in Hong Kong began since June 2019, which was triggered by the Extradition Bill that would have enabled the government to allow extradition of criminal offenders to the People's Republic of China. The persistent protests have been further complicated by COVID-19 outbreak from January 2020.

A local survey with 170 frontline reporters after the exposure to tear gas in July 2019 suggested more than 90% and 70% of survey respondents presented with respiratory and skin problems respectively (2). Another local survey conducted by The Hong Kong College of Psychiatrists interviewed 80 clients who sought for mental support, and found nearly 50% had anxiety symptoms. There were also 40% and 11% of clients presented with depressive symptoms and post-traumatic stress symptoms respectively (3). In addition, a 10-year prospective cohort study focusing on depression and post-traumatic stress showed that the recent "social incident" created a heavy mental health problems which requires much additional social and health services (1).

In general, the younger generation is not optimistic about Hong Kong's future. For example, a survey shows that 90% of young people opposed the Extradition Bill (4). The survey shows that their dissatisfaction mainly stems from distrust of the government and the system, as well as from their thwarted pursuit of democracy and freedom and is not related to housing or economic development issues, as some have claimed. They also feel a lack of support from the older generation. Moreover, generational disagreements about the movement have led to strained family relationships in many cases. University students were more heavily involved in the movement, as evidenced by the serious damage done to two local universities after they were occupied by protestors and police with contamination from tear gas, petroleum bombs, and other chemicals.

While health-care professionals and social workers are trained to be alert to the negative physical and psychiatric problems during and after crises such as social unrest, the identification and management of susceptible individuals are seldom discussed in the local medical and academic field, due mostly to the unexpected and rapid surge in demand for service. In Hong Kong, practical difficulties exist because many affected individuals did not seek professional care (1). Since local surveys have already reported adverse consequences on both physical and mental health, GPs who can manage both the health aspects and be easily accessible in the community, become important resources for individualized treatment. The role of GPs especially in the aftermath, in responding to natural disaster has been well demonstrated in the Queensland flooding in 2019, when the residents and their GPs were the ones who stayed and put their lives back together after the politicians and the emergency rescuers finished their missions at the end of the disaster (5). The GPs in Australia are also working with their Government in supporting the communities affected by the recent bushfire crisis (6).

Health is not simply absence of illness. In fact, it has been regarded as a state of well-being in the physical, mental, spiritual and social domains (7). While the impairment at the physical and mental health levels is more obvious during social unrest, social and spiritual components of health are often neglected in general medical consultations. Yet, these four dimensions of health are equally important in nurturing whole person wellness. Considering that they are interlinked, if GPs can treat patients with such a holistic approach, the overall outcome will surpass the effects of traditional treatment of symptoms or of each component individually and will result in whole person wellness. Medical Humanities scholars and practitioners have put forth the idea for some time now that "understanding the subjective experience of illness as something distinct from the biomedical attribution of disease" as an important health enterprise (8).

Although the prevalence of mental health problems is high in university students, they have hurdles in seeking help (9). Recognizing this issue, a tailor-made "Mental Wellness Clinic" (10,11) under the University Health Service was set up at a local university in 2016. With the ongoing social unrest in Hong Kong, and evidenced by the latest survey (1), it is believed that the mental health of local university students will be of growing concern. Therefore, health professionals should go beyond treating physical symptoms and pay attention to hidden psychological, social and spiritual problems.

Based on the above background, this paper explores the communication micro-skills needed when treating a student with apparent physical symptoms in the GP office at the University Health Service via a case study. The effort of rebuilding whole person wellness is discussed throughout the case study of the ongoing therapeutic process. Ideally, medical consultation is composed of universal scientific evidence as well as culture-bound medical humanities. According to Atkinson et al. (8), "The medical humanities are most frequently thought of as a means of mobilizing the arts and humanities in the context of medical practice and pedagogy". This article draws on the notion and highlights the creative value of the diagnostic and therapeutic process via the four dynamic steps of composition in ancient Chinese poetry: opening (起), elucidation of the theme (承), sublimation (轉), and summing up (合). According to Fan Deji of the Yuan Dynasty, "There are four movements in poetic composition: smooth opening, unhurried development, change of direction and deep conclusion. With reference to this conception and put it within the holistic medical context, this can be translated into "early detection and rapport building" (起), "exploration and management of related psychological issue" (承), "linking with social and family context" (轉), and "spiritual identity" (合). Such an approach enables the GP to develop a sense of empathy and identification with the patient, establish good communication practice, while at the same time instilling in the patient the necessary openness and trust.

OUR STUDY

This study adopts a case study methodology framed by a Medical Humanities approach. Heale and Twycross (12) stated that a case study as "an intensive, systematic investigation of a single individual, group, community or some other unit in which the researcher examines in-depth data relating to several variables". For example, they adopted a case study strategy to examine pediatric pain management amongst nurses. Similarly, Crowe et al. (13) pointed out that "the case study approach allows in-depth, multi-faceted explorations of complex issues in their real-life settings." For example, Yarborough (14) presented a case study to help a patient with diabetes.

The present case study describes the presenting problems of a young patient affected by the recent social unrest and outlines the intervention process (such as what counseling questions were raised) used by the GP. In addition, reflections by the consulting GP (first author) with reference to the available literature on clinical intervention and counseling are highlighted. Following the common practice in qualitative research, we present the findings, observations and reflections together, which is followed by a general discussion section.

Intervention process and reflections

Opening (起): Early detection and rapport building. Peter (P anonym to protect patient confidentiality) is a 20-year old university student presented to a GP in the University Health Service as a walk-in routine appointment.

> GP: "Hi Peter, I'm Dr X. What can I help you today?"
> P: "I have had asthma for years. Within the last month, I have coughed more frequently and sometimes felt shortness of breath. May I get some medicine for my cough?"

At the first juncture, medical assessment should be performed immediately to exclude medical emergency conditions, such as asthmatic attacks, which indicate the need for early medical treatment or even resuscitation for unstable conditions. After a first clinical assessment, Peter's condition was regarded as stable, but he was diagnosed with suboptimal asthma control without regular medical support or drug treatment in the past few months.

> GP: "Peter, your asthma can be better controlled with the inhaler I will prescribe for you today. I will demonstrate how to use it later. However, do you have any idea why your asthma worsened in the past few months?"
> P: "Well, although I have not participated in any frontline protests, my home is in a district where frequent rallies occur. I believe the air quality is very poor because of tear gas contamination. My eyes and throat are often irritated, and my eczema worsened as well."

Handling multiple symptoms in a single medical visit is a common challenge for GPs. If, due to time limit, it is impossible to manage all the symptoms in one, it helps to prioritize them according to urgency and severity, so that those of less concern can be handled in follow-up visits. If the symptoms share a similar pattern, such as in Peter's case, where problems of his airway, eyes and skin are all precipitated and aggravated by chemical irritation, proper medical advice targeting the cause of exacerbation should be given, apart from prescribing symptomatic drug treatment. In times of social unrest, doctors may need to familiarize themselves with some hitherto unexpected medical diagnoses, such as chemical irritation or burn wounds as a result of contact with tear gas, pepper spray, blue dye from water cannon with unknown content, petroleum bombs, or even gun-shot wounds. As medical literature regarding possible short term and long-term consequences from cyanide and dioxin poisoning is limited, GPs are advised to keep updated via continuous medical education and, if in doubt, refer likely patients to specialist care.

GP: "I'm sorry to hear that your home is affected. How are you now? Is there anything else I can do for you?"

P: "Doctor X, can you give me some sleeping pills? I have very poor sleep these days. My brain is so stuck and I just can't concentrate."

A recent study conducted by WHO showed that in 2015, only 16.4% of students with mental disorders received professional help within the twelve months (9). The problem of low help-seeking rate but high prevalence of mental health problems has been a longstanding issue among college students, both globally and locally. Dragojlovic and Broom (15) explained that "Whilst to care for has traditionally been considered virtuous, despite limited recognition as a social act/relation (particularly for women), to be willing to receive care has also been an important dynamic in the landscapes of suffering". Some of the reasons why students (and many other people, for that matter) are unwilling to seek help in the first place are the fears of stigmatization and/or embarrassment about being considered a 'mental patient' (11). The public generally shows difficulty in accepting people with mental illnesses and this is particularly the case for Chinese people (16). While it is relatively easier for patients to voice out their physical symptoms to their GPs, it becomes a golden opportunity for a GP to actively open up the dialogue once the GP can feel if the patient may also suffer from psychological disturbances. This can be done by simply showing care and concern at both verbal and non-verbal aspects during doctor-patient communication when handling the physical symptoms. Once rapport is built after patient can feel the care from the GP, patient will feel comfortable and safe to express their underlying psychological concerns. This is the first step (起) out of the four steps of composition described above: a relaxed opening consultation that consists of responding to the immediate concerns of the patient (i.e., addressing Peter's physical problems including asthma and eczema flare up), showing care to the patient, and establishing a safe environment for the discovery of other related psychological issues.

Elucidation of the theme (承): Exploration and management of underlying psychological concerns

GP: "Being unable to sleep well for months does cause suffering. No wonder you look so tired. Peter, please feel free to tell me more about your sleep."

P: "I try to go to bed at midnight, but I just can't sleep until five in the morning. Doctor X, I have really done my best to close my eyes, but my parents and brother are so noisy. Even if I ignore them, I can feel my heart beating very strong and fast. It's really disturbing."

Based on the responses of 12,000 participants aged 15 years and above, it was found that almost half of them showed sleep disturbance in the past 30 days (17), including "difficulty in falling asleep within 30 minutes?, "intermittent awakenings, or difficulty in maintaining sleep during the night?, and "early morning awakening and unable to sleep again". Shek and Cheung (18) showed that irregular sleep was prevalent in university students. Given that insomnia is such a common problem in the community, GPs must be capable of managing insomnia arising from different causes. There are many causes for insomnia and specified treatment is very important. In Peter's case, his nocturnal cough and itchy skin rashes due to the flare up of his asthma and eczema were accountable for the organic causes of his poor sleep. These symptoms will be eliminated upon better control of his physical problems as mentioned above.

On the other hand, Peter mentioned at least two additional factors contributing to his poor sleep, namely disturbance from his family members and his palpitations. These hints should lead to an exploration of his sleep environment as well as his mental health state. Taking a detailed history of his family and social situation is also indicated. At this juncture, further psychosocial exploration requires time, which is unlikely to be finished within 15 minutes. Hence, given that the GP also has other scheduled patients, he or she needs to decide whether this unplanned extended consultation is feasible. If there is a practical constraint that does not allow the GP to extend the consultation, the GP should use the precious 15 minutes to do a brief mental state examination, focusing on any urgent mental issues such as active suicidal thoughts, self-harm behaviors, or psychotic symptoms. If either of these urgent mental issues are present, for safety reasons, the GP should handle this patient first and triage other patients for later consultations. If no urgent issues are present, the GP should show empathy, acknowledge the suffering from insomnia, reassure the patient that sleep problems can be managed well with regular medical follow-up, and schedule an extended consultation timeslot as soon as possible. Since in this case, Peter presented to University Health Service that has a Mental Wellness Clinic tailor-made for university students in need of longer follow-up appointments, and Peter was referred for further management under the care by the same GP.

Peter, his parents, and his older brother live in public housing. His father, in his late fifties, is a security guard and has been underemployed since he suffered a back injury a few years ago. The mother is in her early fifties and is a waitress with long working hours. Peter's brother is two years older and works a freelance computer job. Peter experienced daily panic attacks, with palpitations, sweating, giddiness and numbness of fingers. He described having an intense fear of death associated with these symptoms, typically reaching a peak within ten minutes. As he could not predict when an attack would appear, and also due to his daytime tiredness as a result of insomnia, he avoided social gatherings and could not continue with his part-time jobs as a waiter and private tutor in the past two months. Since the University had an early term break due to the unrest, Peter had mostly been staying at home. In particular, the frequency of the panic attacks increased after his previous high school classmates told him that one of their classmates committed suicide a month prior. The suicide note suggested a relationship to the social unrest. However, recurrent flashbacks that are usually indicative of post-traumatic stress disorder were absent.

GP: "Peter, have you ever heard of panic disorder?"

P: "Yes, I have read a lot about this on the internet. I have already done an online questionnaire and I think the score is highly suggestive of this panic disorder. I just don't know how to tell other people. I worry others will think that I'm crazy. Doctor X, will I live like this for the rest of my life? Is there any hope that I can recover?"

GP: "Panic disorder is common. Drug treatment and psychotherapy are highly effective for treatment of panic disorder. Peter, we will walk together through the rehabilitation journey in the coming few months. You won't be alone."

For a patient showing mood disturbance, it is necessary to assess suicidal behavior because mental disorders such as depression have the strongest influence on suicide (19). Suicide accounts for 1.5% of all deaths, with approximately 800,000 suicidal deaths every year (20). In 2015, suicide was the second leading cause of death for the 15-29 years age group in the globe (21). The US National Strategy for Suicide Prevention recommends the use of tools to predict suicide (22), and the European Psychiatric Association endorses using these tools as adjuncts to an individual psychiatric assessment (23). However, current evidence of routine use in emergency departments and in primary care is weak (24). Of course, these tools should not replace the clinical judgment of doctors. Suicidal assessment should be incorporated into the entire process of doctor-patient communication, especially since verbal and non-verbal hints can often be subtle.

GP: "I'm sorry to hear that your high school classmate committed suicide a month ago. Have you ever had similar thought?"
P: "I don't have this thought. I just have a strong fear of death during the panic attacks."

GPs should not hesitate to ask about suicidal thoughts because asking suicide did not lead to significant increase in suicidal ideation in the patients (25). GPs should raise their awareness of common predisposing and precipitating factors as risk factors for suicide. During detailed history taking, Peter does not show a strong predisposition, such as family history of suicidal behavior, previous attempts, or adverse childhood experiences. He does not have a history of drug or alcohol abuse. However, during times of social unrest, precipitating factors such as life events and the effects of the media are more common. GPs should maintain high awareness and be confident in performing suicide assessment whenever indicated. Among persons who attempt suicide, 1.6% die by suicide within the next 12 months, and 3.9% die by suicide within the next 5 years (26). If patients admit to suicidal thought or previous attempts, it is vital to consider the following five points in assessing and managing the risk of suicide (27):

1. A person who presents with suicidal thoughts may be at risk for suicide even if there are few overt symptoms of a psychiatric disorder.

2. Suicide risk should be assessed by considering predisposing and precipitating factors, including recent life events.
3. Risk of suicide should be managed through regular follow-up.
4. The suicidal person, family members, and those who provide care should all take part in ensuring a safe environment.
5. If the risk of suicide is considered to be high or uncertain, the person should be referred immediately to mental health services.

Apart from drug prescription, Cognitive Behavioral Therapy (CBT) shows effectiveness in treating panic disorder (28,29). According to the National Collaborating Centre for Mental Health, CBT with 1-2 hours per week for a maximum of four months since commencement is a recommended choice. In Hong Kong, this guideline is often not practical, mostly due to the lack of expertise and busy clinic schedules. For some cases, the patients may have to wait for more than one year before the first consultation session (30). Although there is no waiting time problem if patient seeks help from private psychiatrists, the charge is high with roughly US$260 per session (31). The cost is similar for consultations with private clinical psychologists (32). With roughly 1.4 million of Hong Kong people are living below the poverty line (33), such high consultation fee is basically unaffordable to them. Hence, in view of the practical difficulties regarding specialist referral, GPs are encouraged to be well equipped with basic psychotherapy skills.

Sublimation (轉): Linking the case with family and social dynamics

Peter showed good compliance with drug treatment for asthma, eczema and panic disorder. He was also willing to arrange regular medical follow-up visits. His cough and skin itchiness gradually resolved within two weeks, together with less frequent panic attacks. However, as he suffers from persistent poor sleep, he cannot discontinue the sleeping pills.

GP: "You mentioned that your parents and brother are quite noisy at home. Are your mood and sleep affected by them?"

P: "Definitely yes! Our family, just like Hong Kong society, splits into two camps. My parents are "blue". I support my elder brother. We are "yellow". We, especially my father and brother, quarrel every day." (Note: "Blue" color symbolizes pro-establishment (including government and police) supporters, while "Yellow" color refers to the side of pro-democracy protestors.)

GP: "It sounds to me that the family has different political opinions. How does this disturb the family in everyday life?"

P: "Well, just like watching TV at home.... My parents basically must watch a pro-government local channel. However, this channel news has been criticized for biased coverage and selective censorship for years. My brother asked them to stop watching it, but of course this ended up in big quarrels. You know, we used to watch TV during dinner time every day. Because we can no longer compromise since the start of the social movement in June, we have not had dinner together since then."

GP: "Is having dinner together important to you?"

P: "Sure. It symbolizes union of the family. However, it is getting hopeless now."

GP: "Why?"

P: As the movement goes on, my brother is getting more involved and actively participates in frontline protests. He seldom comes home now. My father strongly believes that all protestors are 'rioters' who made his son walk away from him. He is so angry and blames them during the TV news every day. My mother, on the other hand, is very indifferent to politics. She just wants to have peaceful dinners with her family. I have tried to educate her about freedom, democracy and civil rights, but it's too complicated for her. She shows no interest. Sometimes I'm so angry with her."

GP: "What makes you angry?"

P: "This is stupidity! Our society cannot be civilized because of the stupidity of many people, including my parents. However, they are my parents, my dear parents…. What can I do? My mother is a traditional Chinese woman who always follows her husband despite their marital problems. I have seen her tears since I was a kid. Doctor X, on second thought, I'm not angry with my mother. She is a victim. I'm so mad with myself! I fail to educate her and make her happy. My brother just leaves home for his social responsibility, but I can't! Whenever I think of this, I end up in panic attacks and can't sleep well."

GP: "I see… So now you have figured out the underlying causes for your panic attacks and poor sleep. I can sense an unresolved anger, correct me if I'm wrong."

P: "Yea… Doctor X, you're right. I'm angry."

GP: "Angry towards…?"

P: "The government, my parents, my brother, and myself…"

GP: "I'm all ears."

P: "Well, it's an undeniable fact that many Hong Kong citizens are dissatisfied with the Hong Kong government. Even my father who is obviously "blue" supporting the police, blames the government for its inability to settle the social unrest. And from our "yellow" perspective, I'm of course angry with the police brutality against the protestors, and the government's betrayal of its citizens, failing to bring universal suffrage. Frankly speaking, I have given up reasoning with my parents. They are both unable and unwilling to listen. Doctor X, have you read "Call to Arms" (吶喊), the famous book written by Lu Xun (魯迅)?"

GP: "Yes, I have a vague memory that this book was included in the Chinese literature curriculum in high school? It attacks traditional Confucian beliefs and the hypocrisy of some Chinese characters, doesn't it?"

P: "Exactly. One of the articles says, we all live in an 'iron cage' which symbolizes society. Now the 'iron cage' is on fire, many people, including my parents, are still asleep. I try to wake them up so that we can escape together. Unfortunately, I have failed. They are still sleeping. Ironically, they don't want me to disturb their sleep."

GP: "So now you are unable to 'wake up' your parents, what will you do?"

P: "I will stay with them."
GP: "Why not just run away?"
P: "I love them. I want to protect them. They are getting old. They need a son by their side."
GP: "How about your brother? Do you think he is just running away or is he doing something?"
P: "He is searching for an exit from the 'iron cage'."
GP: "So..."
P: "So that we all can escape, if there is an exit, hopefully..."
GP: "Good to hear the words 'love' and 'hope'."

Summing up (合): Spiritual identity - The last piece of the jigsaw

Hong Kong has a special history tracing back to 1842, when Hong Kong was ceded to the British Empire because of the Opium War. It had been a British colony until 1997. In the Hong Kong Basic Law (34), it is stated that the existing capitalist system and way of life will continue for 50 years since 1997 (i.e., the socialist system will not be practiced in Hong Kong). Besides, individual rights including freedom of speech, press and assembly, are protected under the Basic Law. The education received by Hong Kong students was influenced by the British during the long years of colonization, where British core values such as democracy, the rule of law, good governance and individual liberty were internalized (35).

On the other hand, Confucian thoughts have also played an important role in shaping Chinese behavior, with harmony as a much valued social value in the Chinese culture (36). The importance of harmony can be revealed in the popular sayings "if a family lives in harmony, everything will prosper; a family will wither if there are a lot of quarrels". In the traditional Chinese culture, children were not socialized to inhibit their emotions in social situations (38). There are five cardinal relations ("Wu Lun") in the traditional Chinese society, namely "sovereign-subject", "father-son", "elder-younger brother", "husband-wife", and "friend-

friend" (37). Children were socialized to play their proper roles in these relationships.

When the core values from the West (e.g., individual liberty) clash with some of the traditional Chinese Confucius beliefs, such as obedience to authority in the society and filial piety (to parents or senior family members), family conflict in terms of culture shock emerges (39). One may argue young students in Hong Kong, like Peter, are born after 1997 and should not have received direct influence from the British. However, it is undeniable that Hong Kong is steeped in Western democratic values. Moreover, in the era of information technology, news and information from all over the world is readily available unless there is internet censorship which is not yet present in Hong Kong. Considering the historic and cultural background, Peter's inner conflict is understandable. He was raised in a Chinese family with parents influenced by Confucianism, as well as under the impact of western democratic values from media, school and peers. When these two values are contradictory to each other, for instance, when Peter's father instructed him to cast his vote for the pro-government candidates in the District Council Election due to obedience to authority but Peter opined voting out these candidates in view of the loss of credibility of the current government. Peter, and in fact many youngsters of this age, would open up to the conflicts of cultural expectations from the senior generation and contemporary cries on self-determination of the millennium cohorts. While parent-child conflict in adolescence is universal, there are unique Chinese cultural features. Chinese parents expect obedience of their children and not to confront with the authority in the society (40). This internal struggle as well as the drop in political well-being (41) may cause Peter prone to emotional disturbance, such as anxiety, depression and insomnia. Although medication can alleviate the symptoms, it cannot solve the root-cause of the internal conflict.

GP: "Well, sometimes it is really difficult to choose between obeying one's parents and following own minds. On a scale from zero to ten, with zero meaning absence of own thinking and full obedience to parents, and ten meaning complete self-determination while ignoring the feelings of own parents, where is your brother on the scale?"

P: "Nine, at least..."

GP: "And how about you?"

P: "Err.... I think I'm standing at five."

GP: "Why do you think your brother stands at nine while you are at five?"

P: "Because he is pretty sure that I will stay at five, taking care of our parents, so that he can do more on the frontline, which is of quite high risk. We know that many protesters lost their lives in the past few months, don't we? Frankly, I respect him for what he does for Hong Kong society. I'm not as strong as he is. I will have asthma attacks if I stay in rallies with frequent tear gas attacks. I can't be a burden to others in the battlefield, so I stand at five. I choose a more peaceful and safer way of protest, such as casting my vote to the pro-democratic party in the recent District Council Election, going to the pro-democratic restaurants, and taking care of my parents so that my brother can go further. "

GP: "I hear the word 'choose'. Is it your own choice to stay at five? Or am I correct to say that it is an underlying consensus between you and your brother to remain at your respective positions?"

P: "Oh Doctor X, thanks for pointing it out. I haven't thought about it in the past. Yes, you are correct. I can say that it is a division of labor in the family."

GP: "How do you feel now?"

P: "Previously, I was frustrated because of a strong sense of uselessness. Now I realize that I can contribute to both society and family. I'm more relieved."

GP: "How nice. And please be reassured that the sliding scale is very flexible. Today you choose to stay at five on the scale, but you can always move up and down at different stages."

P: "Sure, Doctor X. I'll remember your words."

Application of the "scaling" technique is commonly used in counseling theories, including Cognitive Behavioral Therapy CBT (42) and solution-focused brief therapy (43). It is a technique of turning a dichotomy into a continuum so that individuals do not see things as "all or nothing". It is used to challenge dichotomous thinking. But how and when to use it is an art. This skill can only be applied effectively if there is a prerequisite empathy and a sensitive exchange between clients and therapists. Moreover, a prior understanding of the client's cultural background can surely enhance empathy. In general, "suffering as a concept challenges our understandings of things, requiring consideration of a series of entrenched dialectics around concreteness versus subjectivities, physicality versus emotionality, externality versus internality" (15).

As mentioned, physical, mental, spiritual and social well-being are intrinsic to the concept of health (7). These four dimensions of health are equally important in maintaining whole person wellness of an individual. As we see in Peter's case, all the four dimensions of health were impaired in the social unrest environment: Physical dimension: Asthma, eczema; Mental dimension: Panic disorder, insomnia; Social dimension: Family conflict, suicide of a former high school classmate; Spiritual dimension: Loss of self-identity and meaning with struggling between traditional Confucius and modern Western values.

In modern Western medicine with its many specialties and sub-specialties, it is not uncommon to see a different expert for each dimension. If we only manage the physical and mental dimensions, the root-causes of the symptoms which originate from the social and spiritual impairment will remain the same. An unresolved root-cause will inevitably lead to a recurrence of the physical and mental symptoms. The Chinese proverb "to cure the symptoms, not the disease" ("治標不治本") perhaps best formulates the essence of such limited treatment. It is important to remember that Peter is a "person" but not "a symptom carrier". The four dimensions of health do not have clear boundaries because they interlink with each other. It is relatively easy to treat each "problem". But bringing the bits and pieces back together and re-establishing a balanced dynamic within an individual is an art. As Franz Kafka said, "To write a prescription is easy, but to come to an understanding with people is hard." Lin and Shek (44) showed that life meaning plays an important role in adolescent well-being. To encourage an individual to search for his or her spiritual identity is like matching the last piece of the jigsaw puzzle. It is of the utmost importance in the regeneration of whole person wellness and helps to "destabilize the distinction between binary notions of health and illness" (15).

GENERAL DISCUSSION AND FURTHER REFLECTIONS

In modern school medicine, it is common for doctors to focus at disease management with reference to international guidelines with strong scientific evidence, such as GINA (45) for asthma and DSM-5 (46) for panic disorder as in Peter's case. However, when it comes to patients with multi-dimensional and interlinking presentations, clinical management should aim beyond disease or symptom management and aspire to attain a patient's holistic wellness. This article is not a protocol or guideline. Rather, it highlights the importance of holistic intervention in form of the related four steps. We argue that intervention in this political context is similar to composing a poem. This is a unique contribution integrating Chinese wisdom and psychological intervention. It can be used as a useful and innovative conceptual framework to guide the overall therapeutic process which transforms from stage to stage which highlights the artful and demanding nature of medical consultation.

There are four major challenges for promotion of holistic well-being among GPs in the local setting. These include time constraint, concern about counseling skills, divergent life values in doctors and patients, and doctors' burnout.

Time constraint

Consultation length in primary care settings vary considerably in the international context. For example, a review showed that doctors spent five minutes or less with their patients in 18 countries (47). In Hong Kong, the average consultation time in general out-patient clinics under the Hospital Authority was about 6.7 minutes in 2008 (48). Although since 2014, the HA has adopted a planning parameter of eight minutes when planning for additional services, time is still a major constraint if patients with multi-dimensional issues, such as Peter, are seen. In Peter's case, the time constraint was resolved because Peter consulted the "Mental Wellness Clinic" of the University Health Service. With the support from nurses and administrative staff, special extended appointments can be arranged. Regarding other general medical services in Hong Kong, the "Integrated Mental Health Programme for Common Mental Disorder Patients in General Outpatient Clinics, IMHP" (49) that was introduced under the Hospital Authority in 2010, is a shared care model involving collaboration between psychiatrists and primary care doctors to help patients with mental disorders. Hopefully, patients with multiple needs can be screened out through short routine consultations and then referred to these extended consultation appointments. Appointment booking in private GP clinics is more flexible because they do not have the same rigid patient quota set by the public or private institutes. Here, at least for those who can afford private care, extended consultation time can be arranged based on individual patient needs.

Concern about counseling skills

Most GPs in Hong Kong are confident in managing physical diseases, such as mild to moderate asthma and eczema in Peter's case. These are bread and butter in daily practice. Some GPs with family medicine training are also competent in treating common mental disorders, such as panic disorder and insomnia in our case study. While drug prescription of common psychiatric medications is an integral part of medical training and can be updated via continuous medical education, the maturation of individual counseling skills can hardly be achieved by counseling lectures or workshops which usually only take up a small portion of the overall medical training. GPs with special interests in counseling do not receive much training in Hong Kong. Only some short-term certificate courses on counseling theory basis without counseling practicum training are available to limited number of GPs at their own cost and time. If individual GPs aim at receiving more in-depth counseling training, such as a structured master course, or regular participation in counseling practicum under supervision by individual experienced mentor, it is usually considered as the GP's own initiative without financial support from central authority. According to local regulations, even if a GP has completed some structured counseling training, such as master of counseling by a local university, the qualifications are not quotable together with the GP's other postgraduate medical qualifications.

Nevertheless, the lack of skills should not prevent the GP from counseling patients in daily practice because research in psychotherapy clearly shows that therapeutic outcomes are only weakly related to theories and techniques of psychotherapy (50). Lambert (51) pointed out that psychotherapy outcomes are attributable to client and extra-therapeutic factors (40%), therapeutic relationship (30%), expectancy and placebo effects (15%) and therapeutic techniques (15%). If we go back to Peter's case, the critical question asked by the GP turning the process from opening (起) to elucidation of theme (承) was "I'm sorry to hear that your home is affected. How are you now? Is there anything else I can do for you?" By active listening, the GP can "hear" that Peter's home was affected by the rallies. Empathy will lead the GP to think that if his home is affected, he will likely need further assistance. For this reason, the GP offered additional help to Peter and did not just prescribe an inhaler. Throughout the consultation process, the only question asked by the GP that can be considered a special "skill" is the application of "scaling", which challenges dichotomous thinking during the latter part of the session. Apart from this, no special skill specific to any counseling theories has been applied. Without doubt, the artful application of certain counseling skills can streamline the entire process and make it more structured. Furthermore, the outcome may be documented more easily. However, showing empathy and utilizing active listening skills should always be the cornerstones for a holistic approach to the patient. Dragojlovic and Broom, in their book "Bodies and suffering" (15) put forth the idea that suffering moves across persons in the therapeutic encounter, and that suffering should not be 'treated' as being contained to the patient [...]. Rather, suffering circulates, rests on different people, and is supported by particular entrenched social relations and roles. Suffering in this context is in fact an assemblage of roles (professional and lay), desires, expertise, fear, dread and hope - all of which are evident within these difficult and important caring relations.

Divergent life values in doctors and patients

While life values rarely matter in brief GP consultations for simple physical ailments, the picture is completely different when counseling involves psychosocial or spiritual issues, issues that increase in times of social unrest. Due to the trust and confidentiality with the doctor-patient relationship, patients will tell doctors about their values towards family, friends as well as political views. As doctors are also members of the same community, they also have their own life values which may or may not be different with their patients. In Peter's case, it might not only be him and the younger generation who suffer from inner conflicts between individual liberty and Confucian beliefs. Doctors who grew up in Hong Kong share the same historic and cultural background and may also experience similar struggles. In times of social unrest, both patients and doctors suffer. However, once a physician takes up the role of a therapist or caregiver, he or she should be non-judgmental and show empathy irrespective of different life values.

For instance, no matter which political view that the doctor and Peter have, they share the same feeling of despair caused by family disharmony and social unrest. Throughout their communication, the doctor neither showed agreement nor disagreement to Peter's political views. In other words, perspectives can vary, but emotions should be genuine, and communication should remain non-judgmental. This is the foundation for rapport building in counseling. It does not always come naturally and might well require some training and experience. If the doctor feels uncomfortable during the consultation process, referral to expertise help should be indicated.

Doctors' burnout

There are three components of burnout, including emotional exhaustion, depersonalization, and reduced personal accomplishment. Medical doctors are prone to burnout, because of their high level of stress in their work (52). In China, burnout symptoms were very high (53). A doctor who experiences burnout may work like a machine at full capacity and becomes unable to feel the emotion of patients, especially in the Chinese community where the expression of emotion can be quite subtle. In this case, it is difficult for a consultation process to progress from the apparent physical level to psychosocial or spiritual levels. The new Chinese translation of "burnout" ("燃竭") further implies exhaustion on a spiritual level (54). While improving the working environment for doctors is important, the promotion of the Medical Humanities may prove crucial for burnout prevention. Besides communication skills, professional judgment and management skills, Medical Humanities also promotes empathy, mutual respect, authenticity, sensitivity of oneself and reflections. Medical Humanities is not "hard skills" which are technical in nature. Instead, it is a process through which "soft skills" are nurtured in doctors through modeling and guidance (53). "Care is, in effect (and in affect), the (somewhat troubled) companion of suffering" (15), and the

Medical Humanities approach can add a humanistic perspective to our understanding of what it feels like to be ill.

Conclusion

People all over the world have the desire to live in peace and harmony, and nurture family life while also striving to fulfill individual life goals. When wars and other unexpected and prolonged social unrest happen, it destroys the peace once taken for granted and causes people of all walks of life immense suffering. This case study illustrated how a university student who presented to the University Health Service with apparent physical symptoms, received care beyond the initial level of disease treatment. After careful screening and conversation, he embarked on a therapeutic process that led to whole person wellness and awareness. It highlights the important role of GPs, especially when dealing with the aftermath of social unrest. This article highlights the importance of a holistic approach to patient treatment, with a special focus on the needs of patients who, in addition to physical symptoms, show signs of mental distress. Although the case study was based only on one person, it is indicative of the general situation in Hong Kong, which suggests the need for a more creative and caring medicine. At the time of writing of this article, and in the midst of the Coronavirus Outbreak, unrests in Hong Kong are flaring up again. It is hoped that all Hong Kong citizens despite different backgrounds and political views can grow and get matured from this social trauma, to be reborn like a phoenix rising from the ashes.

References

[1] Ni M, Yao X, Leung K, Yau C, Leung C, Lun P, et al. Depression and post-traumatic stress during major social unrest in Hong Kong: A 10-year prospective cohort study. Lancet 2020;395(10220):273-84.

[2] Kwong PY. District councillor explaining symptoms of inhaling tear gas. The Stand News 2019. [Chinese]

[3] The Hong Kong College of Psychiatrists. The Hong Kong College of Psychiatrists claiming over 40% showing depression symptoms in hundreds of help cases. Apple Daily 2020. URL: https://hk.news.appledaily.com/local/20200103/ZRW53YZOZCV7VSE2HG767DRBI4/. [Chinese]

[4] Chung R. "Anti-Extradition Bill" Youth Opinion Follow-up Study. Hong Kong Public Opinion Research Institute 2019. URL: https://static1.squarespace.com/static/5cfd1ba6a7117c000170d7aa/t/5df3158f04b7db043c7da1bd/1576211867361/PCF_Anti_Extradition_Bill_Stage+3_rpt_2019dec13_first+edition.pdf.

[5] Clements M. One year on: After the Townsville floods. newsGP 2020. URL: https://www1.racgp.org.au/newsgp/gp-opinion/one-year-on-after-the-townsville-floods.

[6] Nespolon H. Now and into the future: RACGP bushfire response. RACGP 2020. URL: https://www1.racgp.org.au/newsgp/racgp/now-and-into-the-future-racgp-bushfire-response.

[7] World Health Organization. Review of the constitution of the World Health Organization: Report of the executive board special group. Geneva: WHO, 1998.

[8] Atkinson S, Evans B, Woods A, Kearns R. The 'medical' and 'health' in a Critical Medical Humanities. J Med Humanit 2015;36:71-81.

[9] Auerbach R, Alonso J, Axinn W, Cuijpers P, Ebert D, Green J, et al. Mental disorders among college students in the WHO World Mental Health Surveys. Psychol Med 2016;46(14):2955-70.

[10] Lo SM, Wong HC, Lam CY, Shek DTL. Common mental health challenges in a university context in Hong Kong: A study based on a review of medical records. Appl Res Qual Life 2018;15:207-18.

[11] Lo SM, Wong HC, Lam CY, Shek DTL. An innovative multidisciplinary healthcare model in student mental health: Experience in Hong Kong. Appl Res Qual Life 2019 Aug 24. URL: https://link.springer.com/article/10.1007/s11482-019-09770-9.

[12] Heale R, Twycross A. What is a case study? Evid Based Nurs 2017;21(1):7-8.

[13] Crowe S, Cresswell K, Robertson A, Huby G, Avery A, Sheikh A. The case study approach. BMC Med Res Methodol 2011;11(1):100–8. doi: 10.1186/1471-2288-11-100.

[14] Yarborough P. Case study: A patient with type 2 diabetes working with an advanced practice pharmacist to address interacting comorbidities. Diabetes Spectr 2003;16(1):41–48. doi: 10.2337/diaspect.16.1.41.

[15] Dragojlovic A, Broom A. Bodies and suffering: Emotions and relations of care. New York: Routledge, 2018.

[16] Ho E, Au S, Bedford C, Cooper J. Mental health issues for Asians in New Zealand: A literature review. Mental Health Commission. New Zealand: Migration Research Group, University of Waikato, 2003.

[17] Department of Health. Report of Population Health Survey 2014/15. Hong Kong SAR. URL: https://www.chp.gov.hk/en/static/51256.html.

[18] Shek DTL, Cheung B. Developmental issues of university students in Hong Kong. Int J Adolesc Med Health 2013;25(4):345-51.

[19] Chesney E, Goodwin GM, Fazel S. Risks of all-cause and suicide mortality in mental disorders: A meta-review. World Psychiatry 2014;13(2):153-60.

[20] Naghavi M. Global, regional, and national burden of suicide mortality 1990 to 2016: Systematic analysis for the Global Burden of Disease Study 2016. BMJ 2019;364:I94.

[21] World Health Organization. Depression and other common mental disorders: Global health estimates. Geneva: WHO, 2017.

[22] Department of Health and Human Services. 2012 national strategy for suicide prevention: Goals and objectives for action. A report of the US surgeon general and of the national action alliance for suicide prevention. Washington, DC: US Department of Health Human Services, 2012. URL: https://www.ncbi.nlm.nih.gov/books/NBK109917/.

[23] Wasserman D, Rihmer Z, Rujescu D, Sarchiapone M, Sokolowski M, Titelman D, ei al. The European Psychiatric Association (EPA) guidance on suicide treatment and prevention. Eur Psychiatry 2012;14(2):113-36.

[24] Bolton JM, Gunnell D, Turecki G. Suicide risk assessment and intervention in people with mental illness. BMJ 2015;351:h4978.

[25] Dazzi T, Gribble R, Wessley S, Fear NT. Does asking about suicide and related behaviours induce suicidal ideation? What is the evidence? Psychol Med 2014;44(16):3361-3.

[26] Olfson M, Wall M, Wang S, Crystal S, Gerhard T, Blanco C. Suicide following deliberate self-harm. Am J Psychiatry 2017;174(8):765-74.

[27] Fazel S, Runeson B. Suicide. N Engl J Med 2020;382(3):266-74.

[28] American Psychiatric Association. Practice guideline for the treatment of patients with panic disorder. Washington, DC: American Psychiatric Association, 2009.

[29] National Collaborating Center for Mental Health, National Collaborating Center for Primary Care. Generalized anxiety disorder and panic disorder (with or without agoraphobia) in adults. Management in primary, secondary and community care. London: National Institute for Health and Clinical Excellence, 2011.

[30] Hospital Authority. Waiting time for new case booking for specialist outpatient services. Hospital Authority 2019. URL: http://www.ha.org.hk/visitor/ha_visitor_index.asp?Content_ID=214197&Lang=ENG&Dimension=100&Parent_ID=10053.

[31] Hong Kong Medical Association. Hong Kong Medical Association Doctors' Fees Survey 2018. Hong Kong Medical Association 2018. URL: https://www.thkma.org/pressrelease/details/20190125_a1.pdf.

[32] HKPCC. Individual, pre-marriage, marital or family counselling. HKPCC 2020. URL: http://www.hkpcc.hk/v2/en-us/price/.

[33] HKSAR. LCQ7: Consultation time of out-patient services of Hospital Authority. HKSAR 2017. URL: https://www.info.gov.hk/gia/general/201711/01/P2017110100484.htm.

[34] HKSAR. The Basic Law of The Hong Kong Special Administrative Region of The People's Republic of China. HKSAR 2017. URL: https://www.basiclaw.gov.hk/en/basiclawtext/index.html.

[35] UK Government. Guidance on promoting British values in schools. GOV.UK 2020. URL: https://www.gov.uk/government/news/guidance-on-promoting-british-values-in-schools-published.

[36] Shek DTL. The spirituality of the Chinese people: A critical review. In: Bond M, ed. The Oxford Handbook of Chinese Psychology. Hong Kong: Oxford University Press, 2010.

[37] King AYC. The individual and group in Confucianism: A relational perspective. In: Munro DJ, ed. Individualism and holism: Studies in Confucian and Taoist values. Ann Arbor, MI: Center for Chinese Studies, The University of Michigan, 1985.

[38] Shek DTL, Sun RCF. Parenting in Hong Kong: Traditional Chinese cultural roots and contemporary phenomena. In: Selin H, ed. Parenting across cultures: Childrearing, motherhood and fatherhood in non-Western cultures. New York: Springer, 2014:25-38.

[39] Hsu FLK. American and Chinese, two ways of life. New York: Abelard-Schurman, 1952.

[40] Shek DTL, Chan LK. Hong Kong Chinese parents' perceptions of the ideal child. J Psychol 1999;133(3):291-302.

[41] Shek DTL. Protests in Hong Kong (2019-2020): A perspective based on quality of life and well-being. Appl Res Qual Life 2020. doi: 10.1007/s11482-020-09825-2.

[42] Zsolt U. Introduction to cognitive behavior therapy. Semmelweis University 2020. URL: semmelweis.hu/pszichiatria/files/2013/02/cbt.pdf.

[43] Tyrrell M. 3 scaling questions from solution focused therapy. Mark Tyrrell's therapy skills 2020. URL: https://www.unk.com/blog/solution-focused-questions-scaling-in-therapy/.

[44] Lin L, Shek DTL. The influence of meaning in life on adolescents' Hedonic well-being and risk behaviour: Implications for social work. Br J Soc Work 2019;49(1):5-24.

[45] Global Initiative For Asthma. Global strategy for asthma management and prevention. Global initiative for asthma 2019. URL: https://ginasthma.org/wp-content/uploads/2019/06/GINA-2019-main-report-June-2019-wms.pdf.

[46] American Psychiatric Association. Diagnostic and statistical manual of mental disorders (DSM-5). Washington, DC: American Psychiatric Association, 2013.

[47] Irving G, Neves A, Dambha-Miller H, Oishi A, Tagashira H, Verho A, et al. International variations in primary care physician consultation time: A systematic review of 67 countries. BMJ 2017;7(10):e017902.

[48] HKSAR. Press Releases. LCQ7: Consultation time of out-patient services of Hospital Authority 2017. URL: https://www.info.gov.hk/gia/general/201711/01/P2017110100484.htm.

[49] Hospital Authority. HA Convention Masterclass 2, from Integrated Mental Health Programme for Common Mental Disorder Patients in GOPCs. URL: http://www3.ha.org.hk/haconvention/hac2014/proceedings/downloads/MC2.3.pdf.

[50] Hubble MA, Duncan BL, Miller SD. The heart and soul of change: What works in therapy. Washington, DC: American Psychological Association, 1999.

[51] Lambert MJ, Bergin AE. The effectiveness of psychotherapy. In: Bergin AE, Garfield SL, eds. Handbook of psychotherapy and behavior change. New York: John Wiley Sons, 1994.

[52] Maslach C, Jackson SE, Leiter MP. Maslach burnout inventory. Palo Alta: CA: Consulting Psychologists Press, 1996.

[53] Lo D, Wu F, Chan M, Chu R, Li D. A systematic review of burnout among doctors in China: A cultural perspective. Asia Pac Fam Med 2018;17:3.

[54] Lo SM. Burnout of a good doctor. Chin Med Hum 2017;3(3):38-9.

SECTION THREE: ACKNOWLEDGEMENTS

About the Editors

Joav Merrick, MD, MMedSci, DMSc, born and educated in Denmark, is professor of pediatrics, Division of Pediatrics, Hadassah Hebrew University Medical Center, Mt Scopus Campus, Jerusalem, Israel and Kentucky Children's Hospital, University of Kentucky, Lexington, Kentucky United States and professor of public health at the Center for Healthy Development, School of Public Health, Georgia State University, Atlanta, United States, the former medical director of the Health Services, Division for Intellectual and Developmental Disabilities, Ministry of Social Affairs and Social Services, Jerusalem, the founder and director of the National Institute of Child Health and Human Development in Israel. Numerous publications in the field of pediatrics, child health and human development, rehabilitation, intellectual disability, disability, health, welfare, abuse, advocacy, quality of life and prevention. Received the Peter Sabroe Child Award for outstanding work on behalf of Danish Children in 1985 and the International LEGO-Prize ("The Children's Nobel Prize") for an extraordinary contribution towards improvement in child welfare and well-being in 1987. In 2017 appointed a Kentucky Colonel by the Commonwealth of Kentucky, the highest honor the governor can bestow to a person. Email: jmerrick@zahav.net.il.

Mohammed Morad, MD, FRCP, born in Israel and educated in the Czech Republic, Israel and the United Kingdom. Professor of Pediatrics at Kentucky Children's Hospital, University of Kentucky, Lexington, Kentucky, United States and Senior Lecturer at the Family Medicine Department, Community Health Division, Ben Gurion University of the Negev, Beer Sheva, Israel. Director of Yaski Teaching Medical Center, affiliated with Ben Gurion University in the Negev. Head of the Patient Safety Circle, Israel Federation of Family Physicians and Member of the Chamber of Ethics in Israel. Member of the Society of Patient Safety and Risk Management, Life Style Medicine, Pain Management and Rural Health Circle under the Israel Federation of Family Physicians. Lecturer on patient safety at Ben Gurion and Tel Aviv University. Researcher and publications in disability studies, Bedouin health research and patient safety. Received the Medical Director Award 2006 from the medical director of the Ministry of Social Affairs, Jerusalem. FRCP of the Royal College of Phyisicians in Edinburgh and the Royal College of Physicians and Surgeons in Glasgow, United Kingdom. Email: morad62@gmail.com.

About the National Institute of Child Health and Human Development in Israel

The National Institute of Child Health and Human Development (NICHD) in Israel was established in 1998 as a virtual institute under the auspicies of the Medical Director, Ministry of Social Affairs and Social Services in order to function as the research arm for the Office of the Medical Director. In 1998 the National Council for Child Health and Pediatrics, Ministry of Health and in 1999 the Director General and Deputy Director General of the Ministry of Health endorsed the establishment of the NICHD.

Mission

The mission of a National Institute for Child Health and Human Development in Israel is to provide an academic focal point for the scholarly interdisciplinary study of child life, health, public health, welfare, disability, rehabilitation, intellectual disability and related aspects of human development. This mission includes research, teaching, clinical work, information and public service activities in the field of child health and human development.

SERVICE AND ACADEMIC ACTIVITIES

Over the years many activities became focused in the south of Israel due to collaboration with various professionals at the Faculty of Health Sciences (FOHS) at the Ben Gurion University of the Negev (BGU). Since 2000 an affiliation with the Zusman Child Development Center at the Pediatric Division of Soroka University Medical Center has resulted in collaboration around the establishment of the Down Syndrome Clinic at that center. In 2002 a full course on "Disability" was established at the Recanati School for Allied Professions in the Community, FOHS, BGU and in 2005 collaboration was started with the Primary Care Unit of the faculty and disability became part of the master of public health course on "Children and society". In the academic year 2005-2006 a one semester course on "Aging with disability" was started as part of the master of science program in gerontology in our collaboration with the Center for Multidisciplinary Research in Aging. In 2010 collaborations with the Division of Pediatrics, Hadassah Hebrew University Medical Center, Jerusalem, Israel around the National Down Syndrome Center and teaching students and residents about intellectual and developmental disabilities as part of their training at this campus.

RESEARCH ACTIVITIES

The affiliated staff have over the years published work from projects and research activities in this national and international collaboration. In the year 2000 the International Journal of Adolescent Medicine and Health and in 2005 the International Journal on Disability and Human Development of De Gruyter Publishing House (Berlin and New York) were affiliated with the National Institute of Child Health and Human Development. From 2008 also the International Journal of Child Health and Human Development (Nova Science, New York), the International Journal of Child and Adolescent Health (Nova Science) and the Journal of Pain Management (Nova Science) affiliated and from 2009 the International Public Health Journal (Nova Science) and Journal of Alternative Medicine Research (Nova Science). All peer-reviewed international journals.

NATIONAL COLLABORATIONS

Nationally the NICHD works in collaboration with the Faculty of Health Sciences, Ben Gurion University of the Negev; Department of Physical Therapy, Sackler School of Medicine, Tel Aviv University; Autism Center, Assaf HaRofeh Medical Center; National Rett and PKU Centers at Chaim Sheba Medical Center, Tel HaShomer; Department of Physiotherapy, Haifa University; Department of Education, Bar Ilan University, Ramat Gan, Faculty of Social Sciences and Health Sciences; College of Judea and Samaria in Ariel and in 2011 affiliation with Center for Pediatric Chronic Diseases and National Center for Down Syndrome, Department of Pediatrics, Hadassah Hebrew University Medical Center, Mount Scopus Campus, Jerusalem.

INTERNATIONAL COLLABORATIONS

Internationally with the Department of Disability and Human Development, College of Applied Health Sciences, University of Illinois at Chicago; Strong Center for Developmental Disabilities, Golisano Children's Hospital at Strong, University of Rochester School of Medicine and Dentistry, New York; Centre on Intellectual Disabilities, University of Albany, New York; Centre for Chronic Disease Prevention and Control, Health Canada, Ottawa; Chandler Medical Center and Children's Hospital, Kentucky Children's Hospital, Section of Adolescent Medicine, University of Kentucky, Lexington; Chronic Disease Prevention and Control Research Center, Baylor College of Medicine, Houston, Texas; Division of Neuroscience, Department of Psychiatry, Columbia University, New York; Institute for the Study of Disadvantage and Disability, Atlanta; Center for Autism and Related Disorders, Department Psychiatry, Children's Hospital Boston, Boston; Department of Pediatric and Adolescent Medicine, Western Michigan University Homer Stryker MD School of Medicine, Kalamazoo, Michigan, United States; Department of Paediatrics, Child Health and Adolescent Medicine, Children's Hospital at Westmead, Westmead, Australia; International Centre for the Study of Occupational and Mental Health, Düsseldorf, Germany; Centre for Advanced Studies in Nursing, Department of General Practice and Primary Care, University of Aberdeen, Aberdeen, United Kingdom; Quality of Life Research Center, Copenhagen, Denmark; Nordic School of Public Health, Gottenburg, Sweden, Scandinavian Institute of Quality of Working Life, Oslo, Norway; The Department of Applied Social Sciences (APSS) of The Hong Kong Polytechnic University Hong Kong.

TARGETS

Our focus is on research, international collaborations, clinical work, teaching and policy in health, disability and human development and to establish the NICHD as a permanent institute in Israel in order to conduct model research and policy.

Contact

Professor Joav Merrick, MD, MMedSci, DMSc
Director, National Institute of Child Health and Human Development,
Jerusalem, Israel.
E-mail: jmerrick@zahav.net.il

SECTION FOUR: INDEX

INDEX

A

F

G

H

I

L

M

N

O

P

Q

R

S

Y